THE **10** DAY GREEN SMOOTHIE CLEANSE

A SECRET TO HEALTHY LIFE

Lose Up to 15 Pounds Juicing.

Protects from 300 Known Diseases

by

M. William

Table of Contents

INTRODUCTION

I want to congratulate you on downloading this book, "THE 10 DAY GREEN SMOOTHIE CLEANSE – A SECRET TO HEALTHY LIFE".

You would know about the health benefits of Green Smoothies and their impact on detoxification. You would meet surprises on every step of this book. So, give it a good read.

Thanks again for downloading this book!

Chapter 1

What Is A **10** Day Green Smoothie Cleanse?

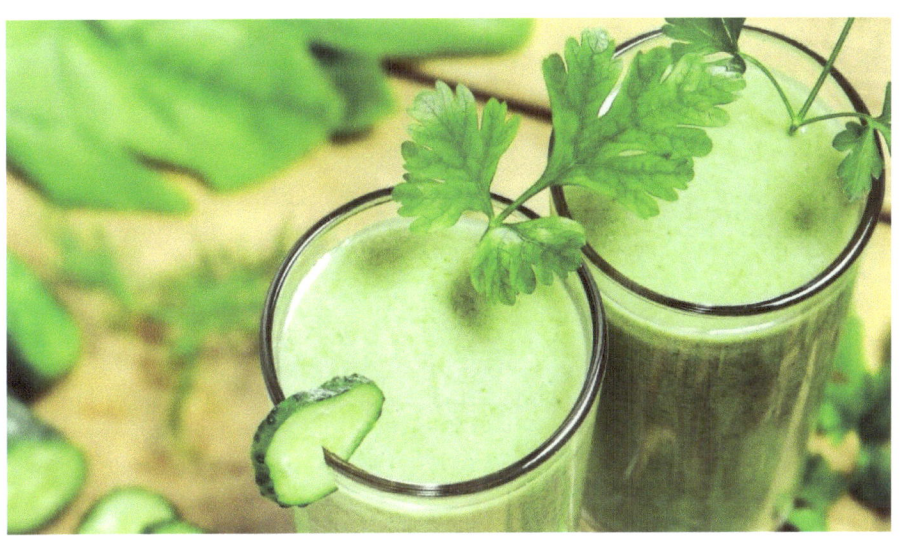

What Is A 10 Day Green Smoothie Cleanse?

Have you ever wondered about the color 'GREEN'? We refer to nature with the word 'GREEN', 'GREEN health' is used for a healthy body similarly 'feeling GREEN' symbolizes freshness of mind and body. So the world GREEN encompasses all the health, nature and freshness in itself. Now imagine a jar full of GREEN, containing all the health and freshness in it and says 'DRINK ME". You are tempted by the fresh green color and take it down your stomach instantly, resulting in an instant current, a 'BiZ' of freshness.

A Green smoothie is a drink in the jar that gives you instant freshness and makes you feel cool simultaneously. The word green itself indicates that it is a mixture of fruits and green leafy vegetables that give boost to the feeling of freshness. It is plant base with additional ingredients which include spinach, kale, collard greens, lettuce and others.

Choosing 'Green' for your health is essentially important as greens symbolize 'nature's blood'. Green itself had been a 'Holy color'. God loves green therefore he covered our earth with a carpet of greens. So, all greens are an essential part of your existences on this planet. You need greens to survive, to feel happy and to CLEANSE yourself and your mind inside out.

Green vegetables carry with them huge packs of nutrients, minerals and vitamins and hence can do wonders to our health. Presence of chlorophyll gives plants their luscious green color and chlorophyll itself gets its pigment and oxygen supply directly from sun. When a food full of chlorophyll enters inside our toxic and worn bodies, it brings healing and freshness along, as maladies thrives only in an environment that is acidic and deprived of oxygen. Hence, Greens can undoubtedly be regarded as our Lifeline.

Greens help us to remove the overload from the body specifically the toxins. For any process to occur inside your body, you first need to detoxify it. Like we first remove the dust from everyday item and then cleanse them using wet mops. Similarly Greens do the essential 'dusting' of the toxins inside the body to make it more adaptive. Detoxification of a body is a must, in order to remain in proper Green health. Thus, the most effective weight loss schedules focus on both fat loss and detoxification, which results in overall improved health. Raw greens are excellent healers. They detoxify your blood plus body by eliminating toxins.

Green Smoothie Cleanse

Every single person in today's world wants a slim healthy body, but it is unfortunate that the food we ingest, the environment we live in, gifts some people with a present of 'obesity'. Every year a huge number of people fall prey to the menace of obesity. Therefore, it calls for a need to take care of ourselves before it is too late for us to revert back. The first step in losing weight is detoxification and green smoothies are the best for the first step of losing weight. Toxins are stored in the fat cells and dieting alone is not helpful in getting rid of them. I present here a little plan of the First step towards losing weight.

One of the major problems in improving the natural health is that people in today's world are so focused on nutrients alone that the true aspect of health is missing. Every breath of air that we inhale, every sip of water that we gulp in, every bite of food, has both good and bad sides to it and our boy is not well equipped to get rid of all bad and to extract all good. So, there is a need for detoxification every time we acquaint our body to new food.

I am sharing here the roadmap for healthy eating that leads to healthy life. This isn't something you do for 10 days and revert back to your old ways. This 10 day green smoothie cleanse is going to transform you in a 'new you'.

Key to health lies in the peace of mind and serenity. You should enjoy whatever you take in and you should feel the consequences as your body gives you signals with every single move you take. So, be confident to raise your mug of green smoothie to your health.

Cheers!

Chapter 2

Why To Use A 10 Day Green Smoothie Cleanse?

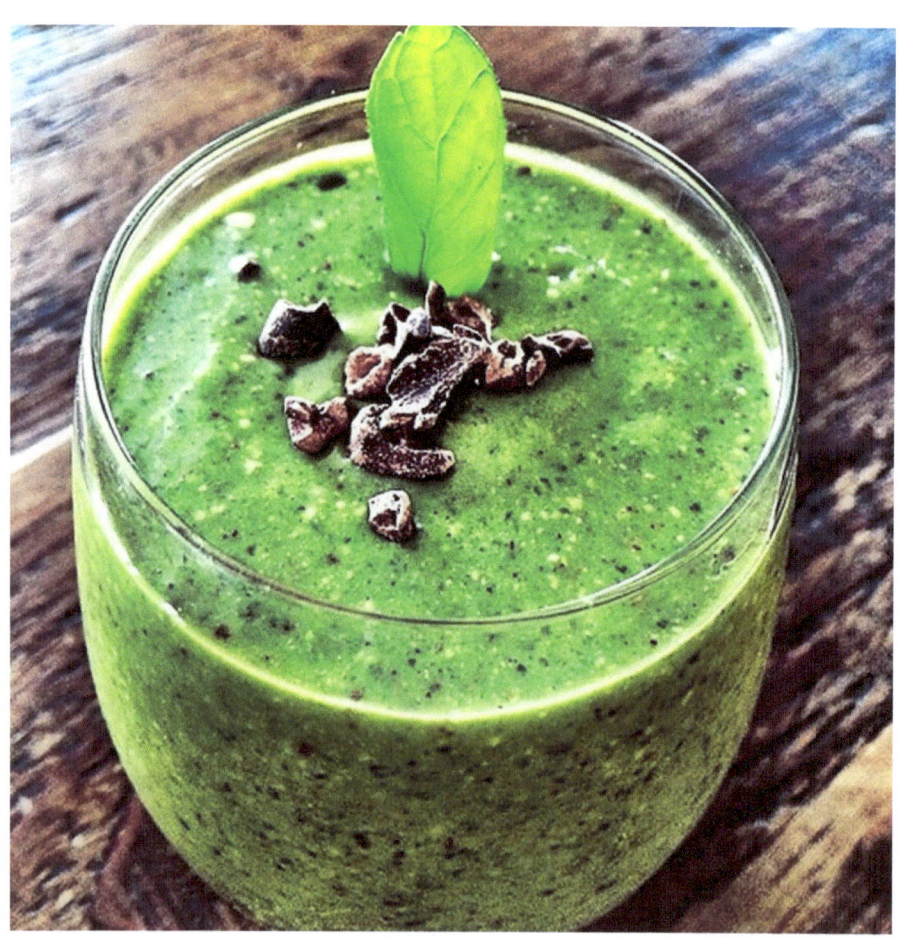

Why To Use A 10 Day Green Smoothie Cleanse?

Focusing on the toxins that are introduced inside our body by the foods we ingest in daily life we need to give ourselves a daily cleansing in order to rid our body of the harmful toxins. We can't avoid eating bananas or other sweet fruits just for the reason that they present us 'sugars' similarly we can't prevent ourselves from ingesting the tempting cream code despite of it containing bulks of caffeine. What we can do is to enjoy things in their 'PROPER' quantities and then getting rid of the bad they might offer.

I today's world, it gets necessary to encourage our own selves to take a step back from the noise of conflicting views about healthy habits and nutrition. We as humans (social animals) need to focus on the big picture of positive aspects of food and nutrition –food, exercise, bulk of water, sunshine and friendship and spending time doing things we love to do. With every breath we take, with every sip of water, with every bit of food we ingest- we expose ourselves to unlimited risks presented by harmful substances they contain. Looking at today's world, it would be no exaggeration to say that 'Detoxification is a key to healthy life'.

Green smoothies offer numerous health benefits. They can include spinach, lettuce, collard greens, parsley, dandelion greens, —any leafy green vegetable in your fridge can participate in the making of a green smoothie but especially those your tongue can enjoy. Here I present a brief introduction to the advantages of Green smoothies made by fruits and green veggies.

Green smoothies offer more health and nutrition than fruit or vegetable juices alone. While extracting juices, we get good amounts of minerals and nutrients but the fiber element is lost. However, smoothies are a combination of whole fruit or vegetables so they offer fiber as well.

Green smoothies account for pure nutrition. The amount of vitamins and nutrients is dependent upon the fruits and vegetables that are used for the smoothie. Most fruits and vegetables have high contents of vitamins specially A and C but certain fruits like Guava have high ratios of folic acid, while avocados provide high amounts of magnesium.

A great way of eating your vegetables is to drink their smoothies. Yes! This is because most of the people like eating fruits and many find it difficult to add veggies in daily routine. Adding fruits to smoothies is a great way to treat your taste buds with the flavor of fruits and at the same time treating you body with the good that vegetables present. Therefore while making smoothies, it is preferred by many to add peaches, bananas or pineapples or whatever one deems tasty.

Smoothies are quick and easy to make. All you need is a blender with a blade and your favorite mug to offer yourself a good date with smoothie.

Green smoothies are also a cheap source of vitamins and nutrients. Why to go for mineral and vitamin supplements when you can get a good amount by ingesting in a mug of Green fresh smoothie.

Children give a tough time to their mums while eating vegetables as most babies are born 'non veg' but Green smoothies present a relief to mums and are a good way to get children to "eat" vegetables. This might need to start with a high proportion of fruits as compared to vegetables but the results would be worth it as they will get used to the taste and will never pose problems while eating veggies.

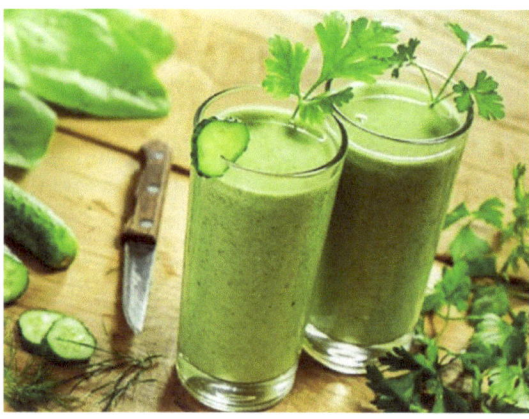 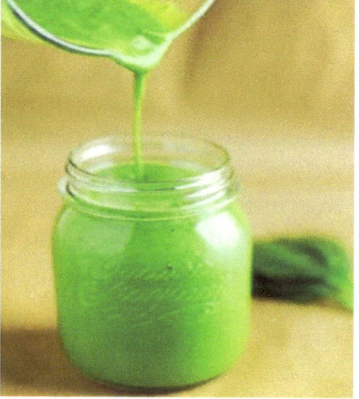

Green smoothies provide with a long lasting source of energy and zeal. Fruits are themselves a good source of energy but eaten along with vegetables would provide long lasting energies as they contain sugars, which do not need long to get metabolized. Balanced sugar content of green smoothies is attributed to the presence of veggies in them.

Green smoothies present low calories. It is a 'wow' thing for all those who want to lose weight. This is because they contain huge amounts of water and fibers that will make your stomach feel full and you won't crave for more food. Thus they help to fight hunger.

As they are already blended, green smoothies are also easy to digest. Your digestive system does not need to work so hard to "break down" the chunks of food in order to extract the nutrients instead the advantages of smoothies will get absorbed as they pass down the gut.

People suffering from indigestion after ingesting a heavy meal will also benefit from green smoothies, as they are rich and light.

Green smoothies will prevent dehydration. Although one needs to drink at least 4 liters of water a day, experts are of the view that most people don't have this much in-take. So, smoothies having huge quantities of water will keep you hydrated for a long period.

In the nutshell, Smoothies can be regarded as a 'Blessing'.

Chapter 3

Getting Prepared

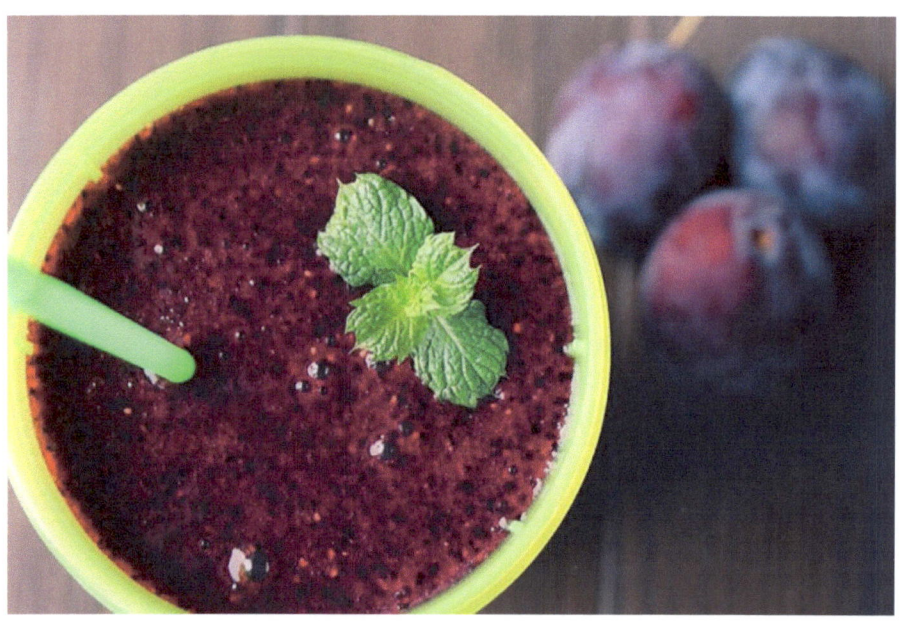

Getting Prepared

Green smoothies are an excellent source of energy and nutrition for those who are planning for a healthy diet. Green smoothies can not only be made part of diet plans but also can be used for daily life. They can be incorporated in daily life as a part of one's meal as well, because they define a 'complete meal'. Those who are planning for a healthy diet plan and incorporating green smoothies in diet need to follow a step by step procedure to enter into the world of Slurping , tasty smoothies.

Step 1

Know yourself, your demands and your favorite flavors. You need to go to some super market to get hold of your favorite fruits and green veggies. All you need is listed as under:

- Recipe cards of green smoothie.
- Standard measuring cups.
- Fruits and green veggies (Washed and dried).
- Plastic bags and jars.
- Marker.

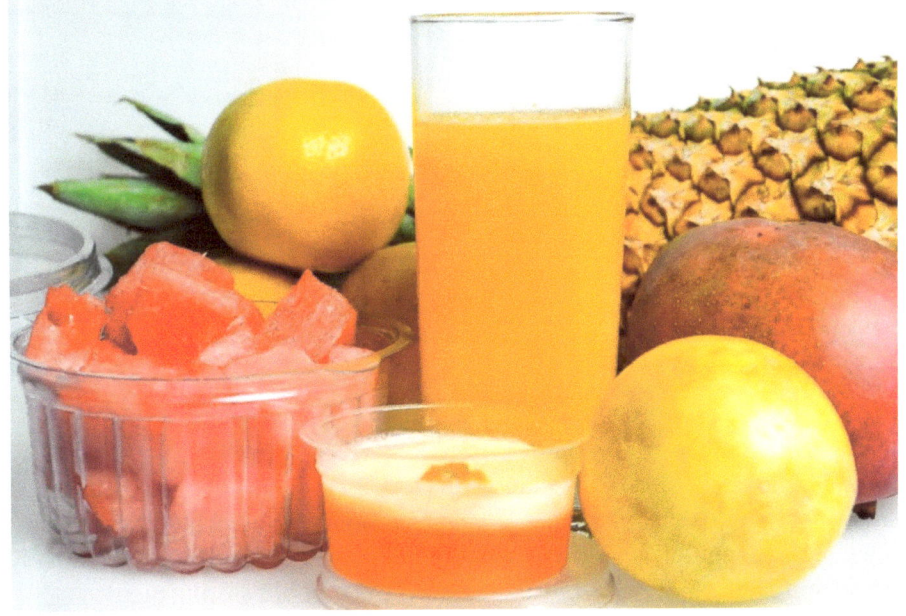

Step 2

Slicing your favorite food into small chunks.

Step 3

Labeling your jars and packets with name and date. You may also need to label the quantities on jars. Labeling jars would help you keeping a detailed and exact account of how much food you need to include in the smoothie according to your recipe card.

Step 4

Measure the quantities and weights and pack them in jars and packets to preserve them in fridge. Remove air from bags and pack fruits and greens in air tight jars.

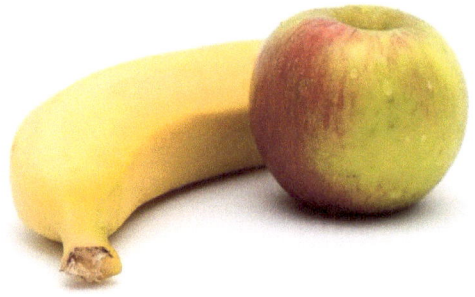

Now you are all ready to prepare your smoothie. Blending your smoothies ahead of time and storing them in sealed jars for 2-3 days in fridge is a nice remedy for busy schedules. But using fresh smoothies every morning has its own perks. Blending smoothies at night and using them in morning is equally good and rather more beneficial as Fresh is the best but storing them beforehand saves a lot of time as cutting food and blending them demands a bit of time.

8 Tips For Preparing Green Smoothies:

1. Take fruits and cut them into smaller pieces and freeze ahead of time in packed jam jars. This will help prevent the fruits and leafy greens from freezing and sticking together in large clumps and thus the smoothies will blend more easily.
2. Thawing the frozen fruits and veggies for a few minutes will lead to smoother smoothies.
3. Store your fruits and vegetables separately.
4. Smoothie packs can be kept for several months in the freezer, but it is highly recommended to use them in best quality within a period of 2-3 weeks (or even lesser).
5. Store your smoothie packs away from foods that have strong odors, e.g. garlic's and onions as you won't want the flavor of fruits masked by that of onions and garlic. Glass jars are the best for this purpose as they offer protection against strong odors and keep fruits in their own best flavors and smell.
6. Smoothies can be blended and kept frozen until they can be used. All you need is to defrost before use.
7. Blend your veggies and add the remaining ingredients and give a nice blend again. Thus creating room for other ingredients.
8. Digestion starts in your mouth so give your taste buds an active start by chewing your smoothie and making your moustache go green.

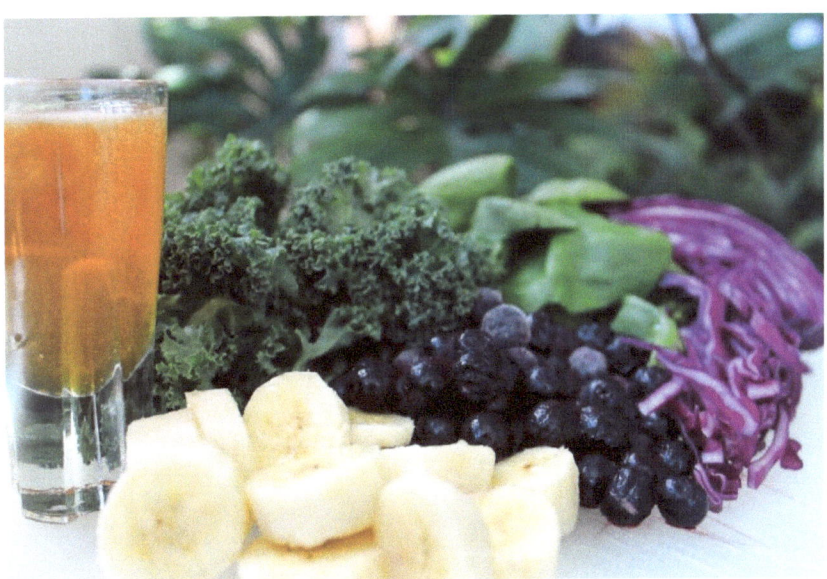

Chapter 4

How To Do A **10** Day Green Smoothie Cleanse?

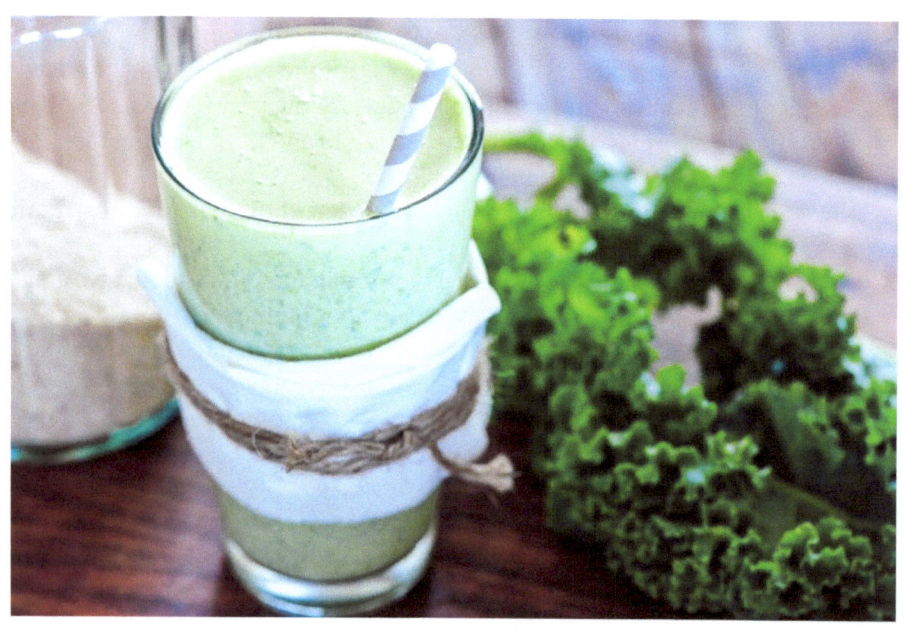

How To Do A 10 Day Green Smoothie Cleanse?

(**Note:** Along with using this smoothie, do ensure that you drink at least 8 glasses of water along with it to ensure detoxification)

Day One

(A smoothie that has more calcium than a glass of milk)

Avoid using dairy products (because they contain fat and might hinder the process of weight loss). Use this smoothie in the morning, after lunch and two hours before going to bed.

- 2-3 cups of Spinach Blend
- 1 cup of orange juice / kiwifruit
- a tablespoon of chia seeds

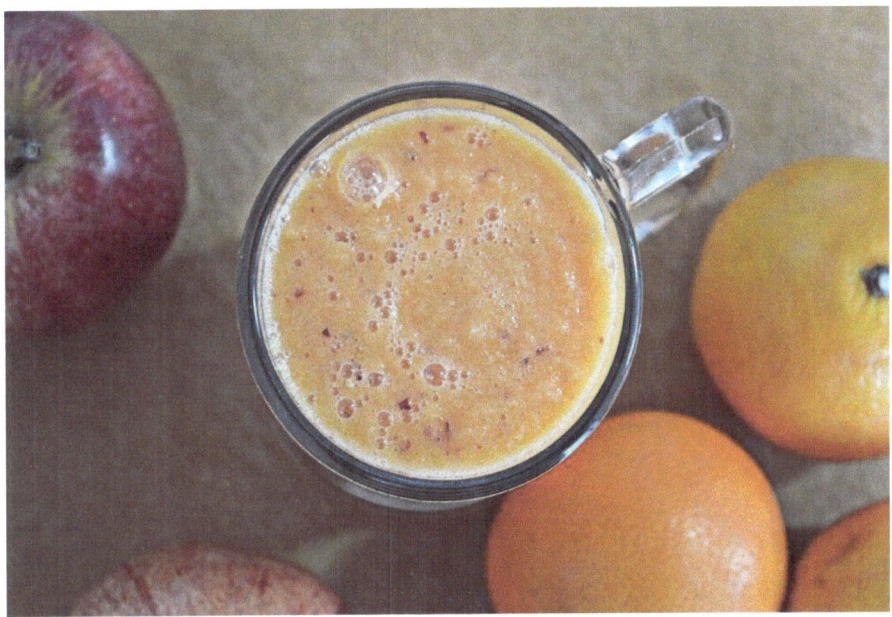

Day Two

(A smoothie that is low in fat)

Avoid using fatty foods and ingest healthy fats like avocados and coconuts. Using a lot of fat will interfere with your body's capability to utilize the carbohydrates and ultimately would lead to weight gain.

- 2-3 cups of Lettuce Blend
- 1 cup of Pineapple juice
- ¼ the cup avocado juice

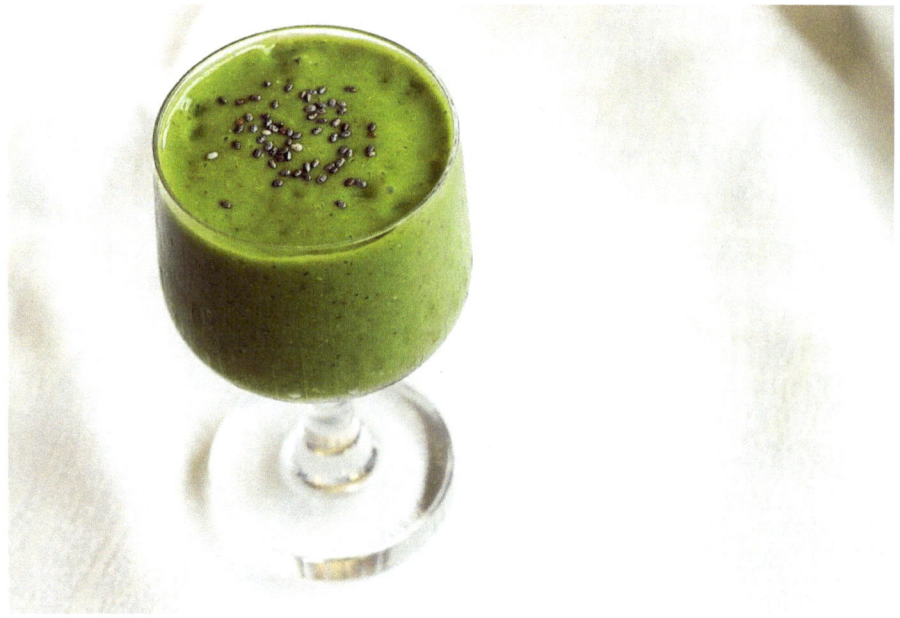

Day Three

(Energy boosting smoothie)

By day 3 some of you might feel like having lost your energy and zeal. So here is the solution to boost your energy up again.

- tbsp cocoa powder
- 1 banana
- 3 cups of Spinach Blend
- Cinnamon

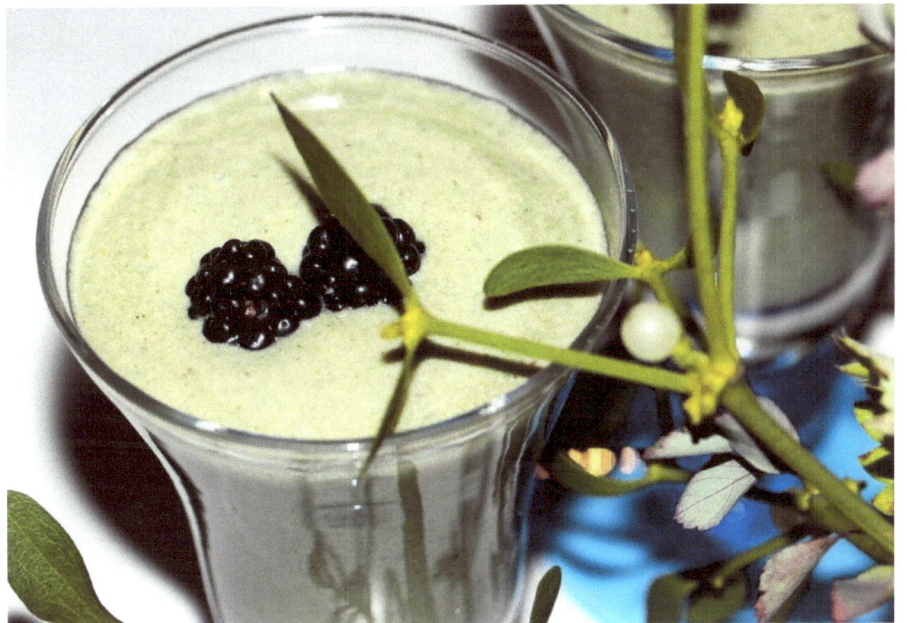

Day Four

(A smoothie rich in vitamin C)

You need to replenish the vitamin content of your body with every day smoothie you take.

- 2 oranges
- 2 cups Lettuce juice
- 1 cup strawberries
- 1 tomato

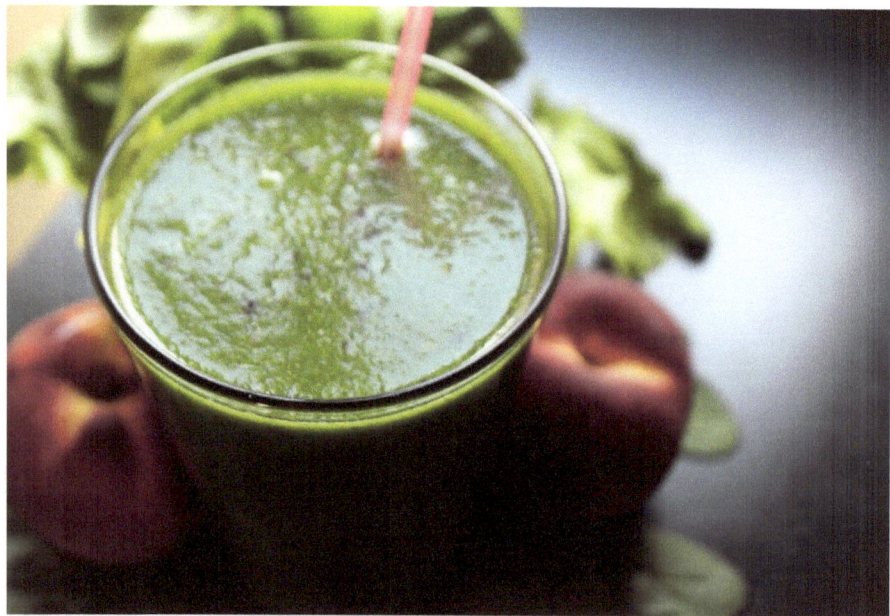

Day Five

(A refreshing smoothie)

When you get bored with the taste of greens, you may want some ingredient that would mask the taste of greens. Cucumber is going to that magic ingredient.

- cup green grapes
- 3 cups of cucumber chopped
- 1/2 cup water
- 1 cup ice cubes

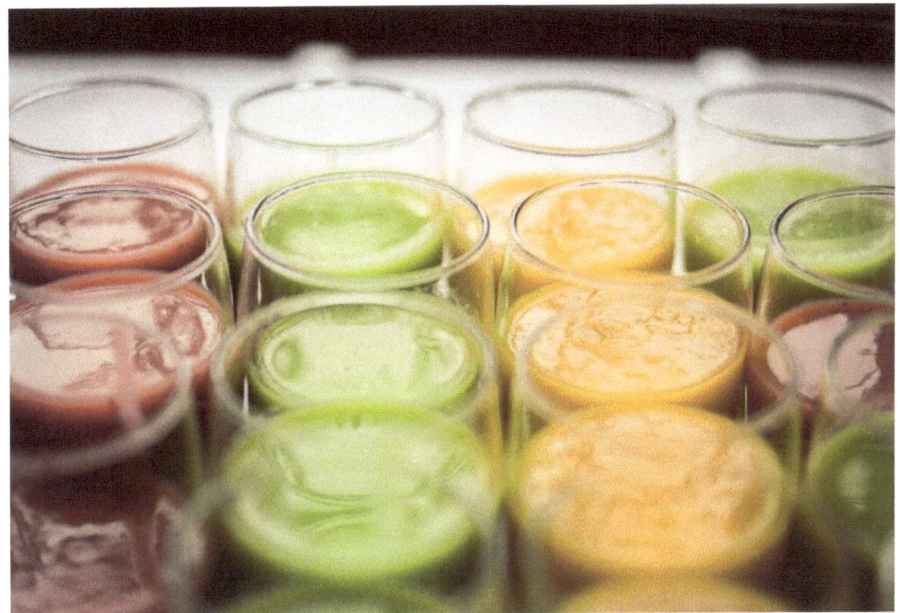

Day Six

(A little sweet smoothie)

Say no to artificial sweeteners instead go for sweet strawberries to add flavor of sweet to your smoothie.

- 2 cups spinach
- 2 cups cucumber
- 1 head of celery
- 3 strawberries
- Juice of 1 lime

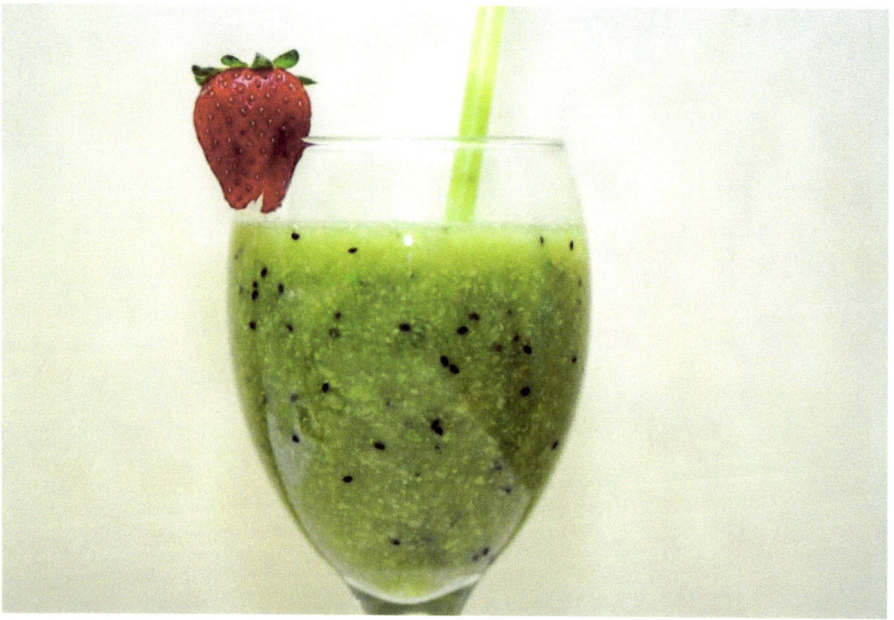

Day Seven

(A highly nutritive smoothie)

Fresh vegetables and fruits are full of fiber, water, and full of micronutrients that boost your metabolism. So instead of using canned food go for fresh greens and fruits.

- 1 head lettuce, chopped
- 3-4 stalks celery
- 1 apple, chopped
- 1 1/2 cups water

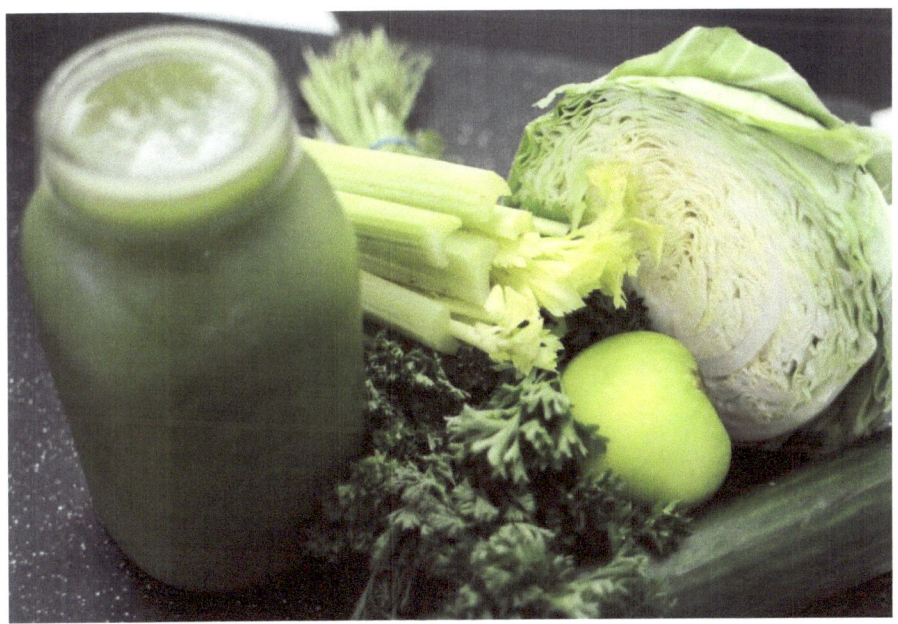

Day Eight

(Your smoothie)

Till day 8, you have had enough of greens so here you need to treat yourself with a little 'No green'. Make a smoothie of your own choice. Add your favorite seasonal fruits and veggies and whatever you like. It's your day Cheers! But wait DONOT, I repeat DONOT add sweeteners, milky products or fattening foods as it might hinder the process of weight loss and you will end up in square one.

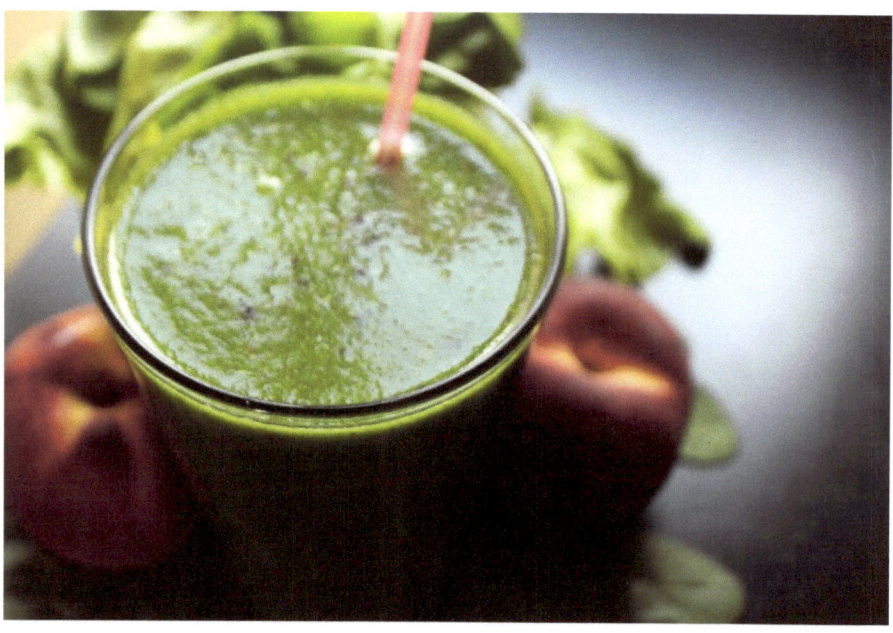

Day Nine

(Break over! back to routine smoothie)

You had your favorite smoothie on Day 8 so here is the time to take some green tea. How about incorporating it in a smoothie?

- 1 cup green tea
- 1/2 avocado
- 1 cup spinach juice
- 1/2 tablespoon Chia seeds
- 1 average sized pear

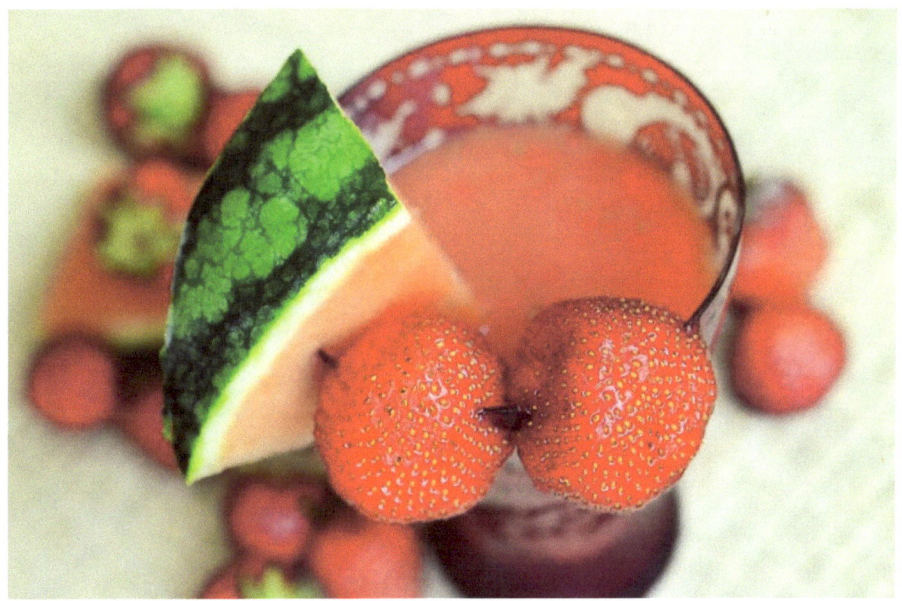

Day Ten

(Happy day smoothie)

It is your 10th day, you have been through a whole 9 days of 'smoothie life' . Congratulations! You did it... Just one more day to go to check how much fat you lost!

- 1/2 cup water
- Mint (a dash)
- Parsley (a dash)
- Barley grass
- 1/4 teaspoon cinnamon
- 1 cup frozen blueberries

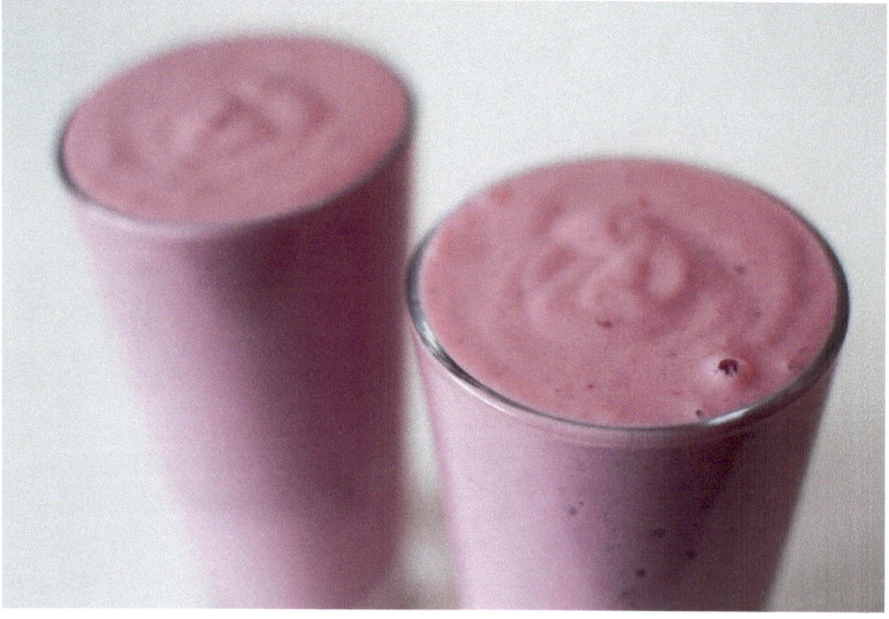

Chapter 5

Tips for Success

Green Smoothie Cleanse

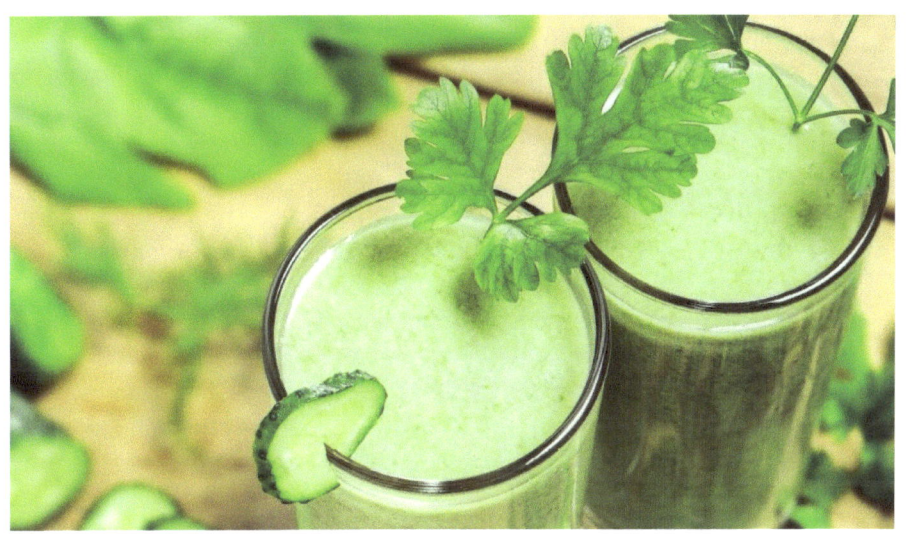

Tips For Success Green Smoothies Cleanse

There are people who go on using Green smoothies without losing a pound. Why is that so??? Probably they aren't making good smoothies. NO! Maybe they don't want to lose weight. I highly doubt that. Probably they aren't following the process nicely. YES! It is because they aren't committed to what they've planned and aren't using the smoothies in their best forms. Here I am presenting a few tips to get the best out of green smoothies in order to lose weight.

- ✓ Start making your smoothies with mild greens, like spinach, and slowly jump towards some intense flavors like parsley. This would help you to get acquainted to the smoothie routine and eventually you'll love incorporating smoothies in your daily routine.
- ✓ Avoid using milk and milk products and make sure that you are using fresh vegetable and fruits to get best results. Milk and milk made products might lead to fat accumulation and you won't benefit from your smoothies in the best way you can.
- ✓ The best experience of taking smoothies is when they are actually 'smooth', without any granules. But you may also find yourself chewing little granules that enter your mouth. Some of you might find it fun chewing them but for other it would be even nicer to first strain your smoothie after getting it blended.
- ✓ Please ensure that you add a bit 'creamy stuff' in your smoothie. Bananas and strawberries add to the creamy mixture of the smoothie. Add creams is an essential part of a smoothie because it would be acceptable to the taste buds and also your stomach would not have to do much effort to mix them all together (makes sense!).
- ✓ Follow your recipes in the start and then refer to those who have used green smoothies. That would help you experimenting with smoothies and adding more valuable ingredients that will surely lead to weight loss. But first know your body as one ingredient that works best for one person might not work good for another. So, know yourself and your demands (a must!).
- ✓ Add colors to your smoothies to make them vibrant and attractive. By adding colors I don't mean to add artificial food colors. Different fruits come with natural appealing colors so you may add strawberries, blue berries, mango chunks etc.
- ✓ Chewing your smoothie is fun but it would be no fun if your find chewable leaves in it so it is better to give a nice blend before pouring your smoothie inside your mouth.

- ✓ There are some people who can't stand warm smoothies so you may also want highly chilled one. I don't recommend adding ice cubes to the smoothies because they would mingle with the texture thus making it thin and no fun. So, it is better to freeze your veggies and fruits before blending them together so that you will have best texture smoothie with enhanced effects and no dilution.
- ✓ There are two methods of making smoothies. One is to mask the flavor of greens by adding your favorite fruits to make it pleasurable to your palate and the second way is to use the greens the way they are. You need to keep on experimenting with flavors so as to make your palate feel all flavors of natural foods. This way you will get best results out of green smoothies you make for your own self. Adding you favorite ingredients will make it easy for you to ingest them.
- ✓ Last but not the least, you need to believe in yourself and your potential, otherwise, you will end up nowhere. Know that if you dream about it you can do it. So, gird up the lion inside you and pave your way to success.

Chapter 6

How To Continue Losing Weight After Cleanse?

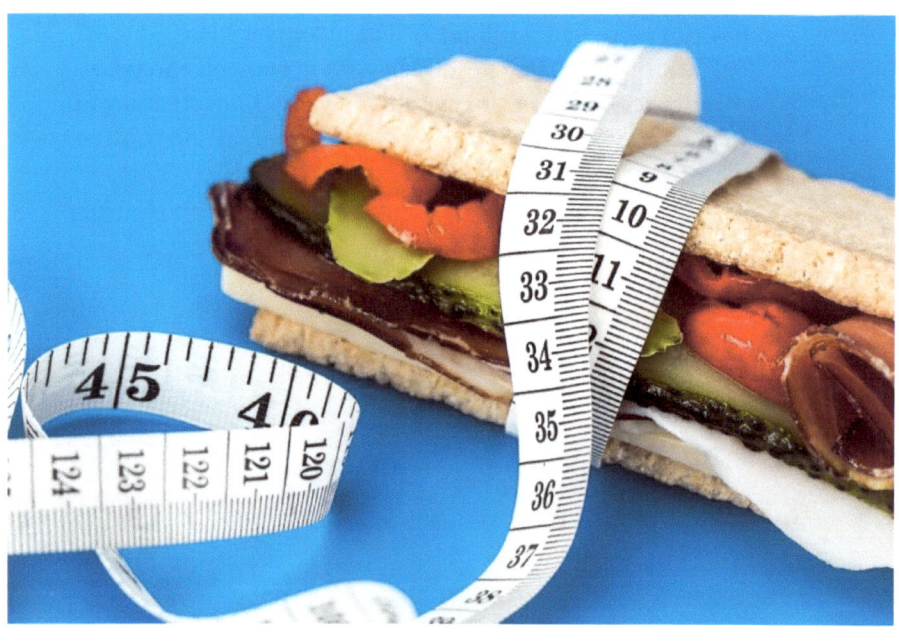

How To Continue Losing Weight After Cleanse?

In order to continue losing weight after the 10 day cleanse, keep taking green smoothies four times a week. In addition to that you will also need to drink a lot of water along with to detoxify your body as much as you can. These methods will bring your hormones in balance and you won't start gaining weight immediately if you follow the routine strictly. I have added a lot of weight loss tips in this chapter and you would gain enough of benefit if you believe in yourself. So there you go!

❖ Incorporate green leafy veggies in your daily diet. , make salads a part of your routine. Take salads before every meal you take. They will boost up your digestion.

❖ Take at least one green smoothie daily and if you cannot take one daily do make sure that you take four smoothies every week with equal intervals in between.

❖ Eliminate calorie foods from your diet instead make low calorie foods a part of your everyday meals. By saying this I don't mean to say that eliminate butters and other fats. Fats make a necessary ingredient of your diet so don't alienate them completely from your life. Take fats but not in amounts that might make you fat as excess of everything is bad so eat as much as you NEED.

❖ Take protein rich foods as much as you can. Proteins along with carbohydrates will give you your boost of energy for the whole day.

❖ Eat less salty and less sugary. Make sure you take in natural salts and sugars as artificial won't do any good to you.

❖ Take white meat instead of red and don't fry your meat. You may just sauté them a bit or adding garlic ginger and olive oil to meat will surely be a plus for you.

❖ An average human needs 20-30 g of fiber per day. So make sure you ingest fiber in goad enough quantity. Fresh fruits and vegetable will provide you with a good share of fiber every day.

❖ Don't restrict your eating times. You may eat whenever you want to. Eat less and eat healthy is the key.

❖ Incorporate organic foods in your diet, drink lots of water and green tea. There is no better detoxifier than water itself so drink as much as you can.

Have A Healthy Weight Loss!

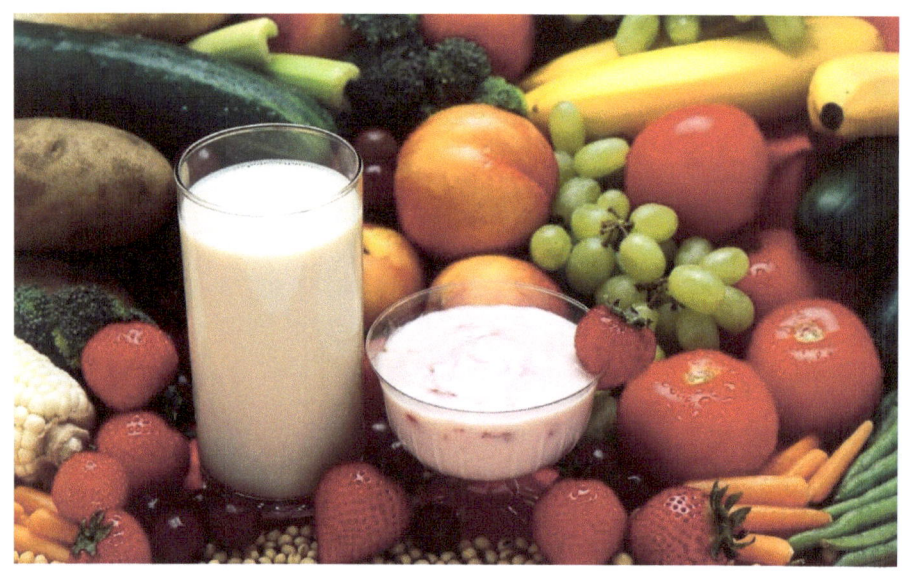

What To Eat For Weight Loss?

Foods To Ingest	Foods To Reject
Animal Protein • Fish – e.g. catfish, cod, flounder, salmon , halibut, herring, haddock, sardines, shrimp, sole, tilapia, trout, tuna • Shellfish and other seafood – e.g. calamari, crabmeat, lobster, oysters	**Animal Protein** • Processed meats like bacon, hot dogs, pepperoni, prime rib, porterhouse
Poultry • hen, chicken, turkey breast, turkey bacon	**Poultry** eggs
Vegetables • leafy greens, asparagus, broccoli, Brussels sprouts, cabbage, cauliflower, celery, cucumbers, collardsgarlic, green beans, kale, lettuce, mushrooms, olives, onions, parsley, radishes, red peppers, squashes, potatoes,	**Vegetables** • Potatoes, corn, and plantains
Fruits • blackberries, blueberries, grapefruits, lemons, limes, passion fruit, raspberries, strawberries	**Fruits** • Canned fruits, fruit snacks
Grains • Barley, Bulgur, Buckwheat, Coconut Flour, Oats, Quinoa,	**Grains** • donuts, white rice, white pasta, white flour
Beans • butter beans, fava beans, garbanzo beans, kidney beans, peas, lentils, navy beans /pinto beans, white beans	**Beans** • Dried beans, fried beans
Dairy • eggs, almond milk, coconut milk, hemp milk, oat milk, rice milk, non-dairy butter	**Dairy** • cheese, cottage cheese, cream cheese, condensed milk, powdered milk, yogurt
Nuts and seeds • almonds, cashews, cedar nuts, hazelnuts, peanuts, pecans, pistachios, seeds: chia seeds, flaxseeds, hemp seeds, pumpkin seeds, sunflower seeds.	**Nuts and seeds** • Sugar-coated nuts
Oils • coconut oil, extra-virgin olive oil, flaxseed oil, sesame oil	**Oils** • Bacon fat , chicken fat, hydrogenated oils (trans fats)
Spices & seasonings • Apple cider vinegar, cardamom, chili peppers, cilantro, cinnamon, parsley, garlic, nutmeg, oregano, rosemary, sage, saffron,thyme, turmeric	**Spices & seasonings** • Ketchup, table salt, mayonnaise, MSG, Worcestershire sauce
Snacks • fruits & veggies, popcorn, unsweetened peanut butter , organic unsweetened chocolate, nuts and seeds, yogurt	**Snacks** • pies, corn chips, cookies, cakes, ice cream pastries, potato chips
Beverages • alkaline water, coconut water, juices, green tea, black tea, mint tea	**Beverages** • Sodas , sports drinks, mixed drinks, beer

More Tips:

Most of the people use juices as weight management tool, but they might return to gaining weight because simple juices have high content of sugars and no fiber in them. Ingest less fiber will hinder in the process of weight loss. If you are searching for a long lasting solution good exercise along with ingesting fresh juices will do no harm. Say yes to the fresh!

People often are too lazy to plan out things for them both before and after cleanse. You need to plan out things to give yourself most of the positive effects. Do not enter into rash eating after cleanse. Go slow, eat slow, Re introduce yourself to foods slowly. You have just been through hard work don't spoil your efforts by jumping in to old routine instantaneously. Above all your mind set is the most important thing. If you see yourself fitting into old clothes when you were slimmer then you will be able to get your slimmer look back but if you go with the flow without dreaming any better you would end up nowhere.

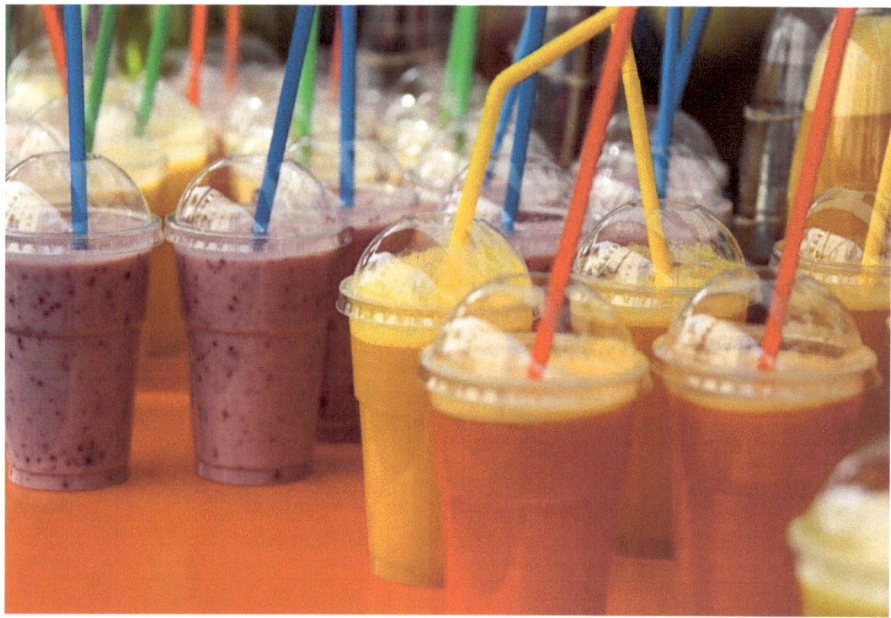

Parents tell their children from early age to eat to their fill and not more than that so if you the golden rules of eating you would not ver gain unhealthy weight and if you are, you need to mend your eating habits. Playing with your foods is one of the best ways to know yourself. The recipes of granny work into play only when you know how to incorporate those old recipes in your new world. Reduce carvings and make sure to ingest just as much as you need or even less. This reminds me of a story of a king who used to ingest foods through both hands, not caring about the amounts. He was so fat that two horses were needed to bear his weight while going from place to place. Once he happened to pass from a field where a young energetic farmer was harvesting the crops. The king saw him and wished to have his energy. He stopped by an end to the farmer to ask 'how do you manage to be this energetic. I am a king, I eat a lot of good food but I don't have a dash of your energy'. The farmer replied ' let me tell you a golden rule. I eat only when I am hungry and never ingest food even if I am presented with manno salwa (the best of foods).

Hence, we all need to eat mindfully.

Chapter 7

Five Detox Methods To Enhance Your Cleanse

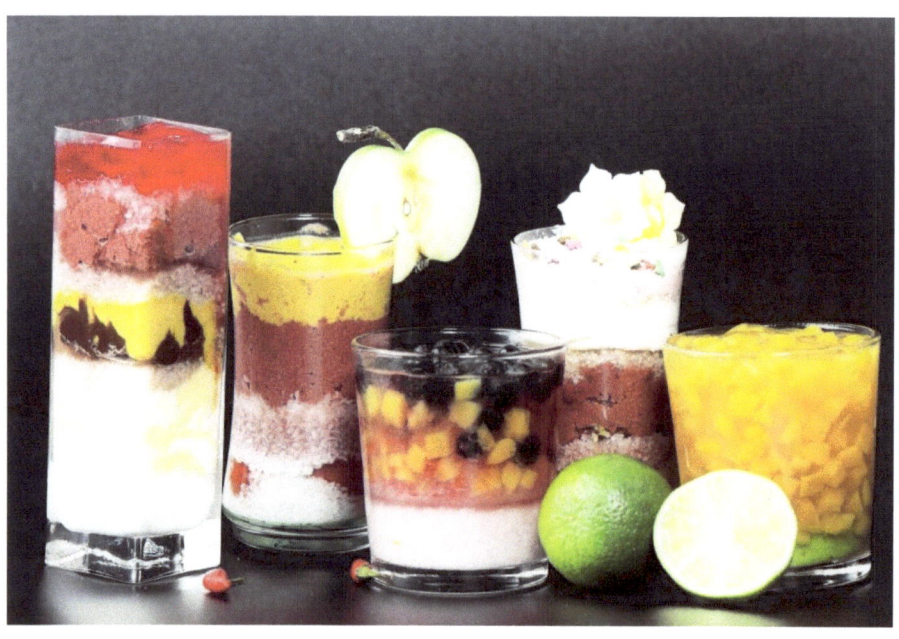

Five detox methods to enhance your cleanse

Detoxification is the process of cleaning the blood. The process occurs by eliminating impurities from the blood inside the liver. Kidneys, intestines, lungs, lymph and skin also help in the process of detoxification. When the impurities aren't properly eliminated, the cells of the body are adversely affected. Every day our body is exposed to all kinds of toxins that present danger to our selves. In order to rid our bodies of toxic agents we need to cleanse our inner systems. Toxins make you feel sluggish and after detoxification you will have your boost of energy back again. Here, I have included five different approaches to consider for losing weight.

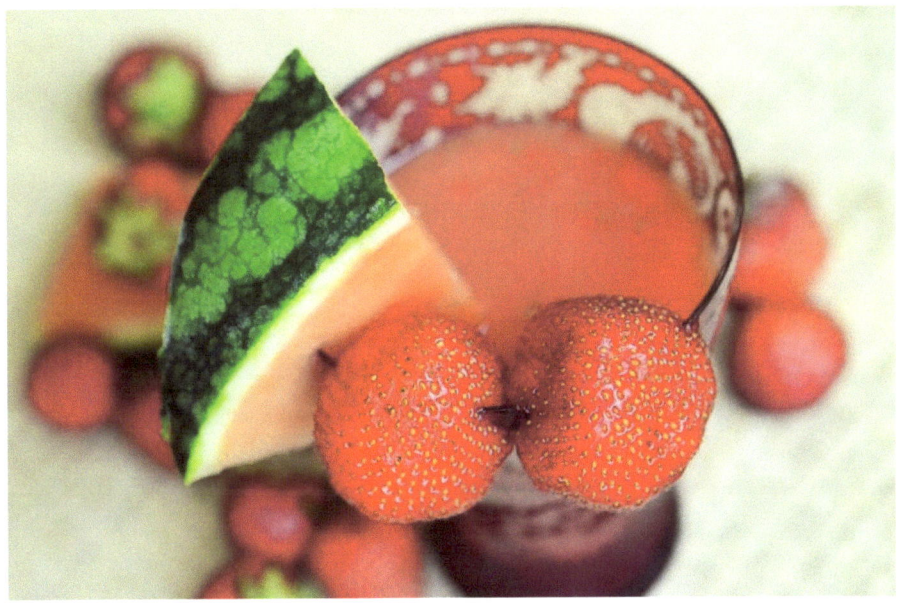

1. Cleanse With Salt

Salt removes bacteria from the lungs and also helps to heal your body. It has been medicinally in order to treat asthma and allergies and inflammation. You will have your internal cleanse through smoothies while for complete detoxification you will also need to work externally. Include salt in your tub (a pinch or two would do) and take a bath with the salty water. You can't prevent yourself from feeling fresh after the bath. Don't use artificial salts. Instead, opt for the natural alternatives. You may also start practicing hydrotherapy by taking a very hot shower for five minutes, followed with cold water for 30 seconds. Doing this three times will transform you into a fresh you.

2. Cleanse With Juices

Intake of juices will alleviate your laziness and will lead to detoxification of toxins from your body thus leaving it fresh and energetic. Incorporate as much greens in your juices as you can. Incorporating fruits in your juices is also a nice tip to get rid of un anted toxins as juices will wipe them out of your body.

Plenty of fiber obtained from fresh fruits and vegetables like Beets, radishes, cabbage, broccoli, spirulina and weeda are excellent detoxifying agents.

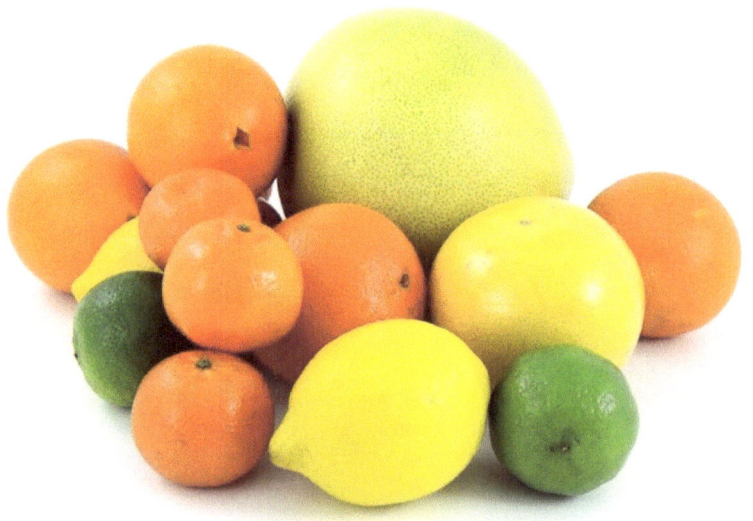

3. Cleanse With Lemon

Lemons are acidic that allows them to aid the process of detoxification. Adding lemons to water every morning and drinking a glass or two will help to eliminate the toxins that accumulate while you sleep. Lemons will also help to degrade fats inside the body hence speeding the process of weight loss. Lemons also help in resetting your body's hormones and neurotransmitters.

4. Cleanse With Exercise

This may also be referred to as 'sweat cleanse'. It is one of the great ways to lose weight and detoxification. Keeping your body hydrated is very important during the process because if you don't keep it hydrated the solutes would accumulate more and more.

Losing weight is a matter of losing fats while balancing energy and nutrition. Exercising triggers the process of weight loss and also activates enzymes and hormones to give their best. You would have to work out to fit into your old jeans.

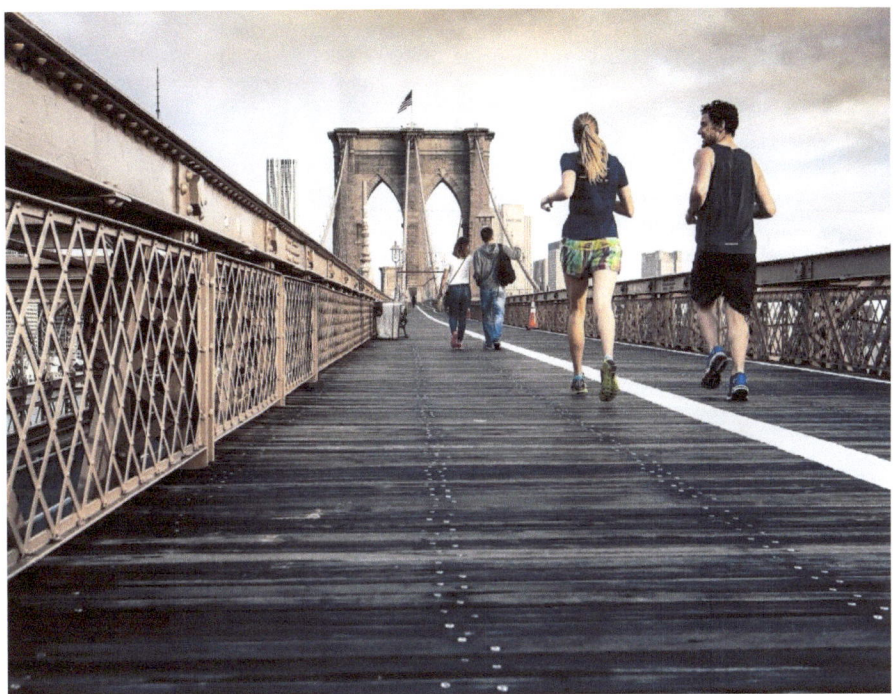

Sweat causes your body to eliminate wastes through perspiration.

The most important way to detoxify is Exercise. One hour every day exercise will provide you with your desired detox results.

5. Cleanse The Lymphatic System

Massaging is one of the most efficient ways of cleansing as it would lead to expulsion of toxins out of the lymphatic system and ultimately out of the body.

Chapter 8

Frequently Asked Questions

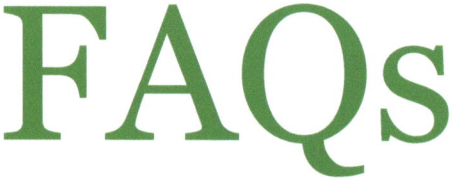

Frequently Asked Questions (FAQs)

Here is a list of few questions about green smoothies and weight loss.

Is it possible to drink too many green smoothies?

Green smoothies present a lot of fiber and add to the nutritive value of your diet. It is important to notice that while talking about green smoothies we have used the term 'incorporate' green smoothies in your diet so it is equally essential to ingest meat and whole grains alongside. As smoothies will provide you with the nutrition from fruits and vegetables but your body will also demand nutrition from other sources as well. So it would be no wrong to say that don't DEPEND yourself wholly n solely on green smoothies but keep experimenting with your food. And taking as many green smoothies as you want won't do any harm to you.

Can I take my daily diet along with using Green smoothies?

Green smoothies themselves present you with a complete diet if you include the ingredients that offer you all the necessary nutrients needed by your body. I won't recommend ingesting high amounts of fat, carbohydrates and proteins but if you make sure to take Proper balanced amounts of these nutrients you may take other foods along with using green smoothies. While taking extra foods keep in mind the dos and don'ts that I have mentioned in this e-book.

Is it necessary to take the seasonal fruits and vegetables only?

No you can play with your ingredients the way you want. Adding seasonal fruits is the best because you would have to go for canned or preserved veggies and fruits. Canned foods do not present as much benefit as natural foods do. So, it is highly preferable to go for natural if you want desired results.

I can't drink 8 glasses of water regularly. How to compensate for it?

Water being colorless and tasteless but it adds all flavors and colors to our life. It is a 'Must' to take 8-12 glasses of water on regular basis. Smoothies present a good alternative to drinking water. You can dilute your smoothies to high water content thus every cell of your body won't be deprived of its share of water.

Is taking green smoothie healthy in pregnancy?

Why not ! Green smoothies will provide you with strength and freshness during pregnancy. You would be able to perform everyday tasks like you did before pregnancy. You can exercise, you can dance and you can do whatever you will. So, don't take pregnancy like a malady, instead welcome your new life with open arms and start to dream about the little feet.

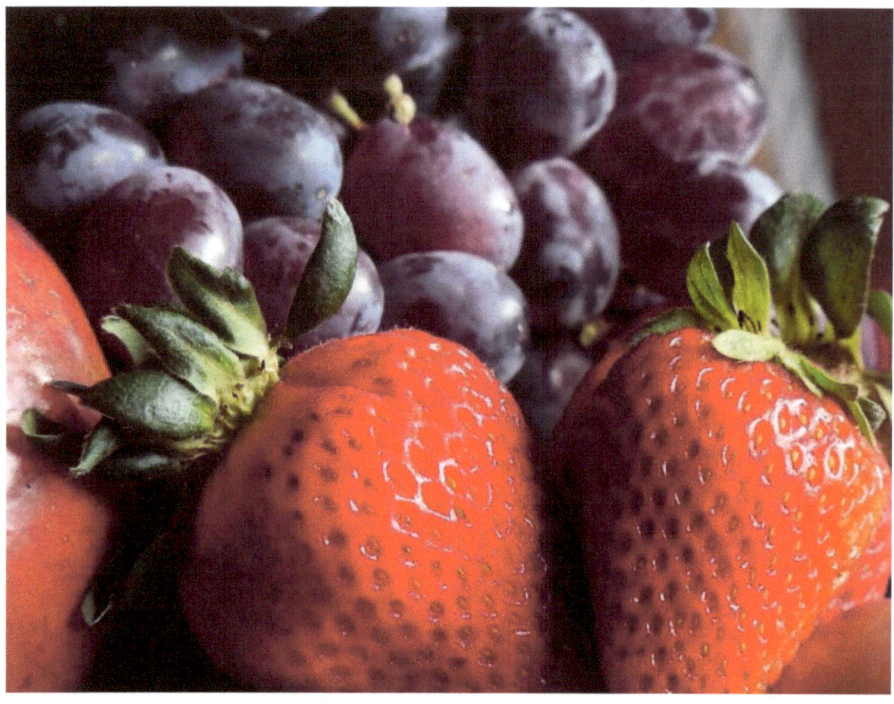

Can I stop taking green smoothies after fitting in my favorite jeans?

By the time you'll fit into your favorite clothes you'll fall in love with the green smoothies. They would have become an integral part of your life by then. So what's the point in switching away from them? Green smoothies is not a 'diet plan', it's actually one way to groom yourself. Green smoothies define a lifestyle which is healthy and cool. So you may keep on using green smoothies after losing pounds because they provide no harm but do wonders to your health. Though you will lose weight but you will have to keep your hormones and enzymes in balance and for that instead of taking pills you can just ingest a glass of a slurping fresh Green smoothie. I recommend using green smoothies four times a week after losing weight. You may incorporate ingredients liked by your palate to keep yourself in shape.

Are green smoothies a supplement of fresh juices?

Not at all, they are even better than the fresh juices. Why? Because green smoothies contain all the fiber of veggies and fruits but fresh juices give you water, minerals and no fiber. You make the best use of fruits and vegetables when you take smoothies. A human body needs 20-30g of fiber everyday and fresh juices do not provide you with fiber. Hence smoothies provide a better alternative to the fresh juices as they replenish your body with essential fiber it needs.

How can I keep my veggies and fruits fresh for longer period of time?

 Green smoothies remain fresh in the refrigerator for 2 days maximum, but some ingredients will surely be lost while refrigerating them. Water may also start to separate. Fresh is the best, you don't have to keep fruits and veggies in refrigerator for long.

How much is a bunch of green vegetables?

A bunch of leafy greens, refers to the one purchased from market as such– for example several leaves of lettuce, dandelion or Swiss chard bundled the way they are. Typically it makes about 3 cups of chopped greens. A bunch can also be referred to an entire large head of broccoli, spinach etc. I generally recommend using 3- 4 cups of greens in a smoothie that you can take for a whole day. 3-4 cups of greens is exactly perfect for one day of smoothie routine.

Why shouldn't I add milk and yogurt to my smoothies?

I don't recommend adding dairy products to smoothies because adding milk, creams and yogurt might hinder in the process of losing weight as they offer a lot of fat. Milky products don't facilitate detoxification of body and won't enhance the nutritive value of other added ingredients. Adding ingredients that add to other nutrients is the key to making good smoothie that is effective in losing weight.

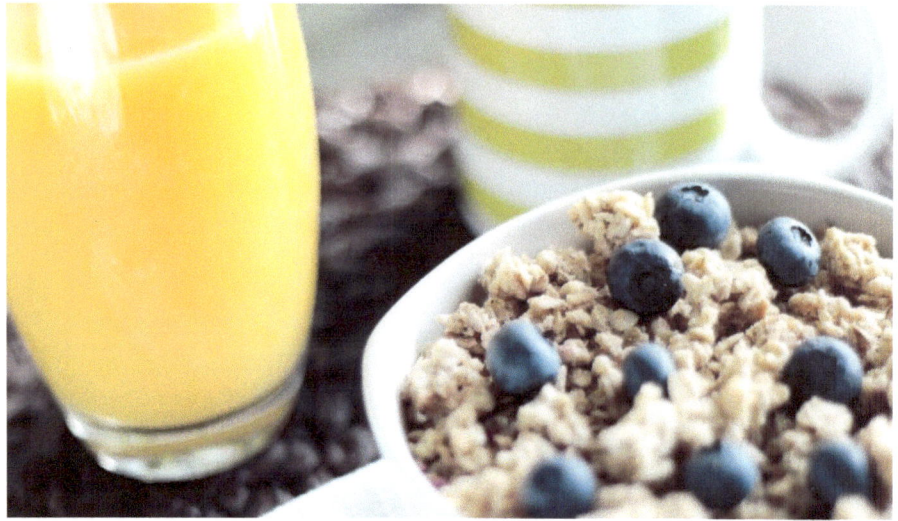

Why do you feel gas after taking smoothie?

Your stomach gives you signals and might be extremely low in digestive acids. Gas indicates that your stomach is trying to get healthy. If you feel some strange symptoms you can reduce the amounts of greens successively.

Green smoothies..

Your way to a better living

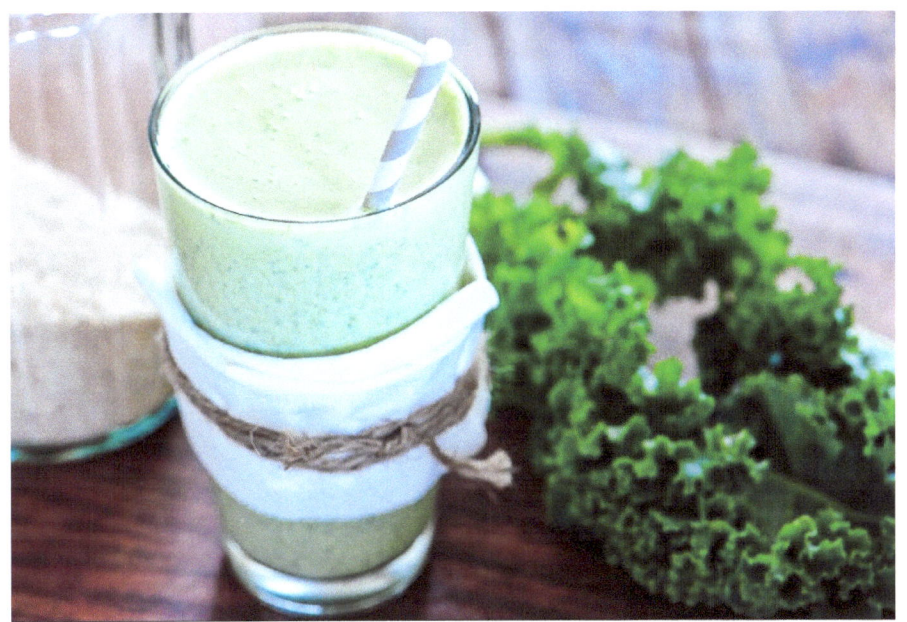

****

Chapter 9

Testimonials

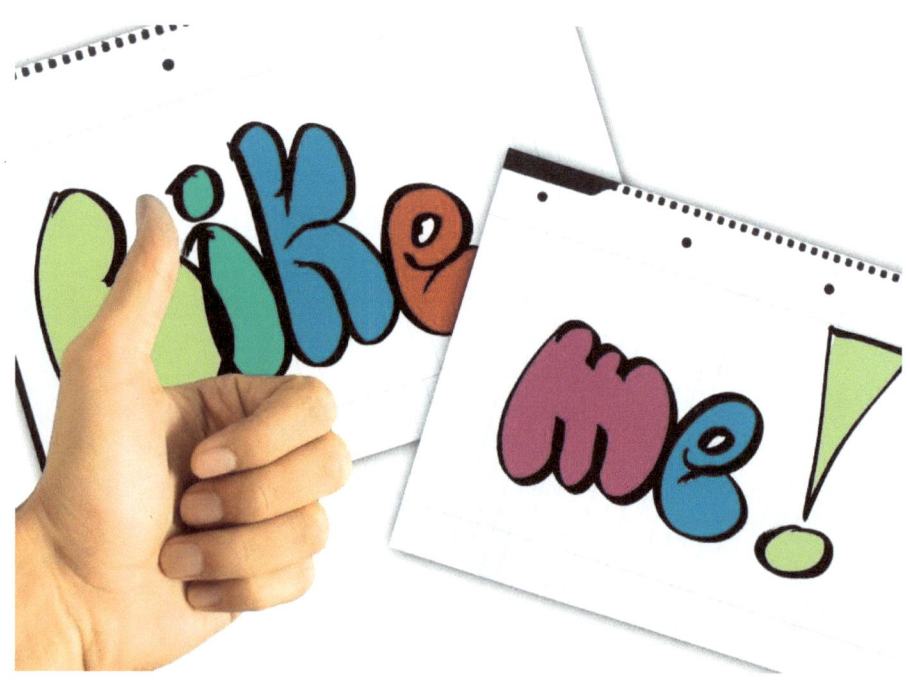

Testimonials

- ✓ I had a few skin problems for which I had to take to take antibiotics and blood cleaners. I started taking green smoothies as remedies and the results were astonishing. My skin started to glow fresher with every week. Now, I have incorporated green smoothies in my everyday routine and I feel happy having greens around me.

- ✓ I started making green smoothies for my husband while he was suffering from indigestion problems and the results were exactly the way I had desired. His problem vanished away.

- ✓ I was 101 kg while I got diagnosed with kidney ailments. The doctor asked me to lose weight to speed up the treatment. I started taking pills and went on crash diet but I ended up nowhere. One of my neighbors told me about green smoothies and their health effects, I thought of giving it a shot. After a month of using green smoothies and regular exercise I lost 30kgs and my kidney treatment went all fine. Now I owe this life to the fresh green smoothies.

- ✓ It is so possible to get addicted to green smoothies. Ever since I got introduced to green smoothies I can't imagine my daily routine without greens. I have decided to make green smoothies my daily routine meal. I love the way I feel after taking green smoothies into my daily diet. Even my family asked about my 10 day green smoothie's recipes and my children love using them daily.

- ✓ I crave for green smoothies when I don't take them for a meal. They have become an important part of my diet. I go regularly to the market to get myself fresh greens and I have been transformed into more energetic person than I was before.

- ✓ I was initially intrigued by the idea of drinking my greens. I used to eat lots of fruits and vegetables but I was looking for an easy way to take my fiber. I love green smoothies and I feel better, thinner and fresher. The combination of green smoothies and lots of water help in weight loss. Now I am more prepared to meet the demands and challenges of my busy days.

- ✓ As a mother I was highly concerned about the diet of my children and family. My family has been drinking green smoothies for the last 2 months since I incorporated greens in my daily routine. I feel an improved overall health. My children were crazy behind snacks and had no love for fruits but now they love the greens I provide them because I make sure to add the ingredients they love. I make fun smoothies for them that keep them energetic for the day. My most favorite's ingredient for smoothies is frozen strawberries.

✓ My husband had a bone marrow transplant and we were very conscious about his nutrition. After using green smoothies he has started feeling healthy and fresh. I can now nurse my child for a longer period as green smoothies have enhanced the quantity of milk in my breast.

✓ I'm 36 years old. I always had regular cycles. But a couple of years ago I started to miss my period for a month or two and it started happening on regular intervals. I got concerned and incorporated green accidently. After about two months of using green smoothies, I returned to a very regular cycle of 20 – 30 days .I've been drinking green smoothie per day for six months now and my cycles are consistently regular. I owe this new health to green smoothies.

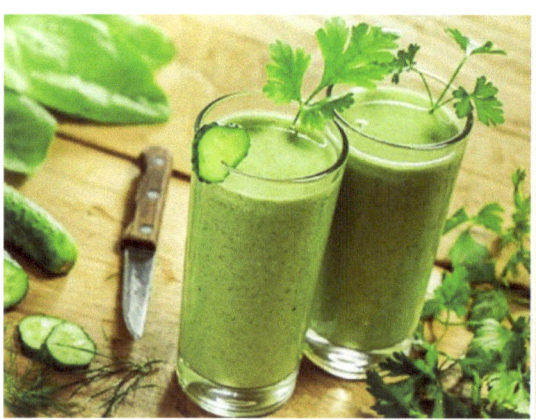
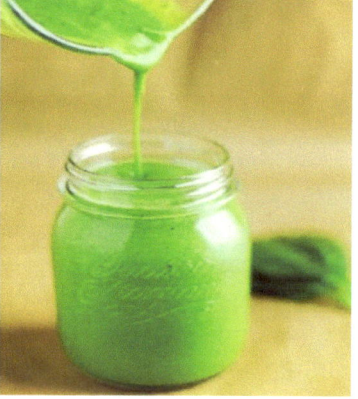

Chapter 10

Green Smoothie Success Stories

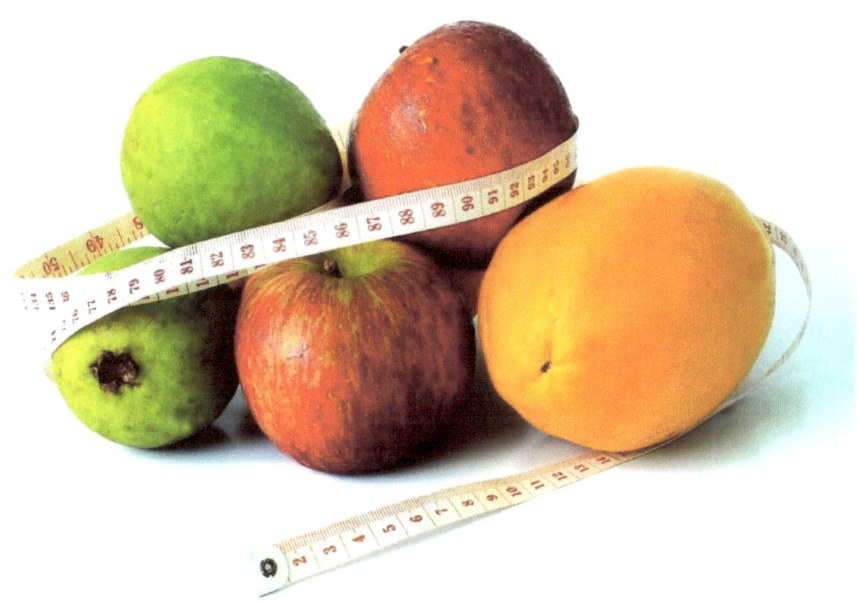

Green Smoothie Success stories

Emily - 34

As a young girl I never loved eating vegetables. A nice dinner to me was a good piece of chicken and a few nuggets. I like taking fruits and juices but said a big no for veggies.

By the time I reached my early 20s, I was bullied for being overweight. My colleagues used to refer me as 'fatty'. I tried a variety of diets and supplements but I was never able to stick to them for long period because I always failed to get the results I was looking for. Once I stopped dieting, I switched back to being overweight. I got married at 26 and starts gaining even more after my honey moon. A friend of mine then introduced me to green smoothies to get into shape and feel good about myself because I felt down after when my husband used to say 'why so fat?'. I started using green smoothies and losing weight afterwards was like a miracle. I kept on using smoothies and doing work outs and now nobody believes I am the same fat Emily from school. I have 2 kinds now and they are proud to tell fellow kids that their mum looks hot and fresh even while managing house hold.

Thank you greens for bringing happiness back to me!

Ayan – 17

My parents met an accident when I was 15. And afterwards they started feeling sick with every passing day. The declining health of my mother and father used to kill me deep inside. I incorporated greens in their diet to get them back to bloom.

After a few weeks of drinking green smoothies my parents started to love them. I brought a more refining blender to my home to make better smoothies. Our green smoothies have become greener and better. Summer is an easier time to drink smoothies due to the warmer weather. However, I manage to maintain using them in winters as well. I don't push my children into drinking smoothies but as they themselves love to ingest fresh foods, they love smoothies too. They have helped me to control my sugar cravings and boosted my energy.

Thank you the 10 day green smoothies!

Success and Happy for Green Smoothie! ... ^_^

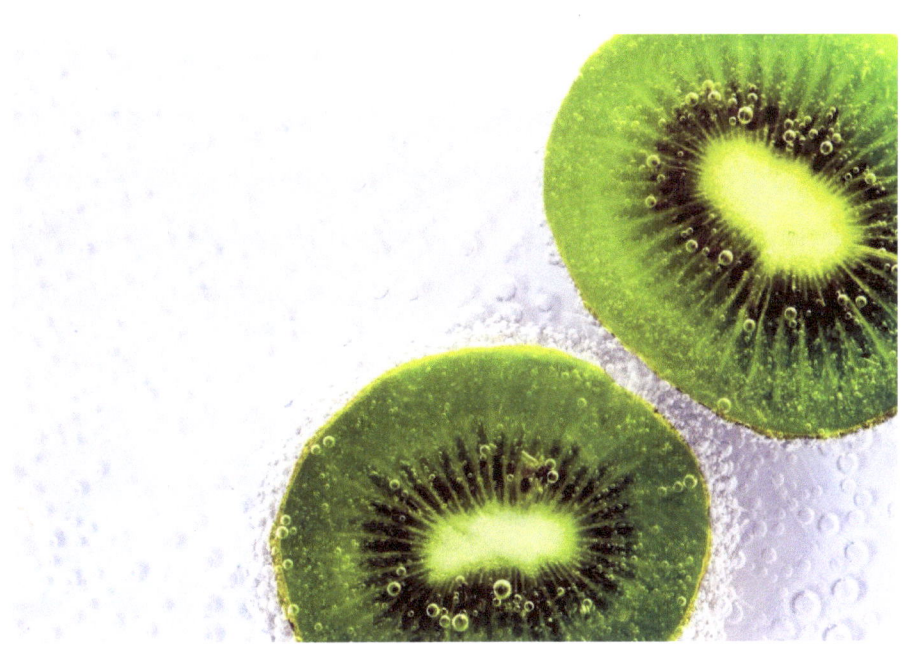

Cheers!

Bonus!

Green Smoothies Recipes for Beginners

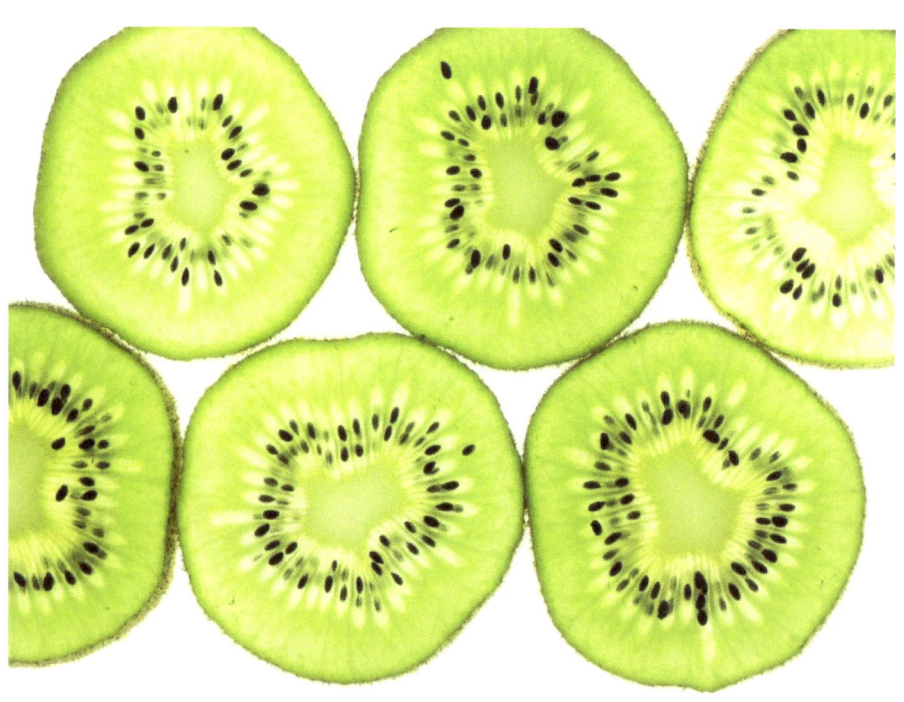

Green Smoothies Recipes for Beginners

Yogurt Based Beginner Smoothie

Handful of spinach, crushed

- 1 cup ripe mangoes, sliced
- 2 tablespoon greek yogurt
- 1 cup sweet pineapple, sliced into medium sizes
- 1 cup of water
- handful of fresh mint leaves

Add together all ingredients into the blender. A few more water and yogurt may be added depending on your desired creaminess or consistency.

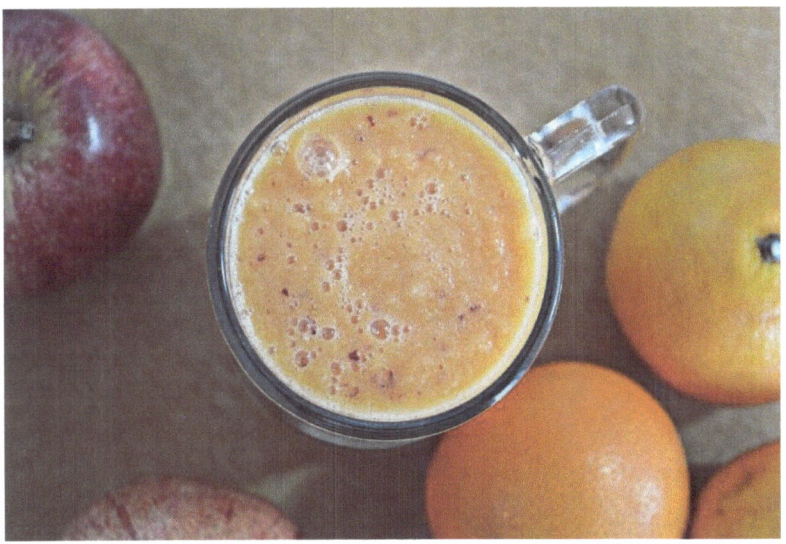

Pineapple Kale Avocado Smoothie

- 1/3 cup fresh pineapple, sliced into chunks
- 1 cup ice cubes
- 1 scoop protein powder
- ½ cup ripe avocado, peeled and sliced
- 2 cups kale leaves
- 2/3 cup vanilla almond milk

Mix all ingredients together in the blender until smooth.

Minty Honeydew Smoothie

- 1-2 leaves fresh mint
- 1 cup ice
- ½ cup coconut milk
- ½ honeydew melon, sliced
- 1 teaspoon fresh lemon juice
- Dash of honey

Jumble all ingredients in the blender. You can opt to garnish smoothie with mint leaves when serving.

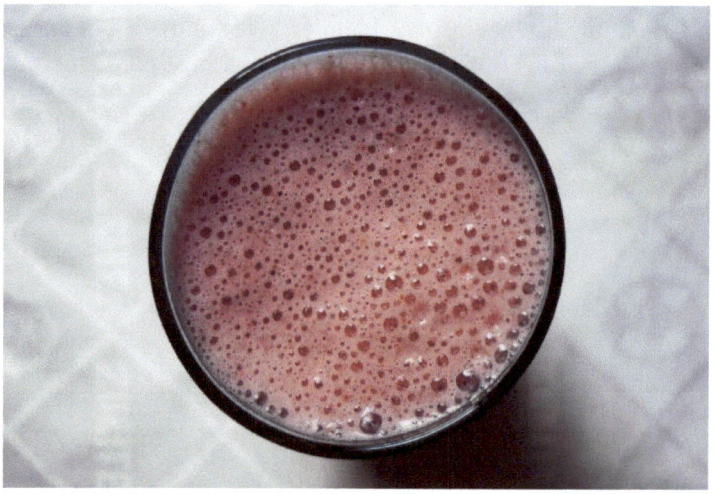

Pineapple Peach Green Smoothie

- ½ banana, sliced
- 1 tablespoon flaxseed
- 2 cups kale leaves
- 1 cup almond milk
- ½ cup fresh pineapple, sliced in chunks
- 1 cup fresh or frozen peaches
- 1 scoop protein powder

Mix all ingredients together in the blender until smooth.

Green Blueberry Smoothie

- 3 cups spinach,
- ½ banana, sliced
- 3 tablespoon hemp protein
- 3 leaves kale
- 3 peaches, sliced
- ¼ cup coconut water
- handful of water
- handful small ice cubes

Blend all ingredients together then add all liquids and ice.

Dandy Green Smoothie

- 1 bunch of dandelion greens, chopped
- 1 banana, chopped
- 2 large apples, peeled and chopped
- 2 teaspoon flax seeds
- handful of spinach leaves
- 1 lemon, peeled and chopped

Blend all ingredients with enough water to cover ingredients.

Kale Strawberry Goddess Juice

- 2 cups spinach leaves, chopped
- 2 apples, unpeeled and chopped
- a handful of fresh mint leaves
- a handful of ginger
- 8 kale leaves, chopped
- 1 lemon, unpeeled and chopped
- 12 fresh strawberries

Mix all ingredients together in the blender until smooth.

Delish Basil, Lime, Cucumber, Apple Juice

- 1 lemon, unpeeled and chopped
- 1 cup basil leaves
- 1 medium size cucumber, chopped
- 2 apples (green or red depending on your preference for a color mix)

Mix all ingredients together in the blender until smooth.

Green Sweet Minty Juice

- ¼ cantaloupe, peeled and sliced
- 2 grapefruit juice
- 1 tablespoon coconut sugar
- 2 mint leaves
- 5 fresh basil sprigs
- 1 cup cold water

Mix all ingredients into the juicer until smooth.

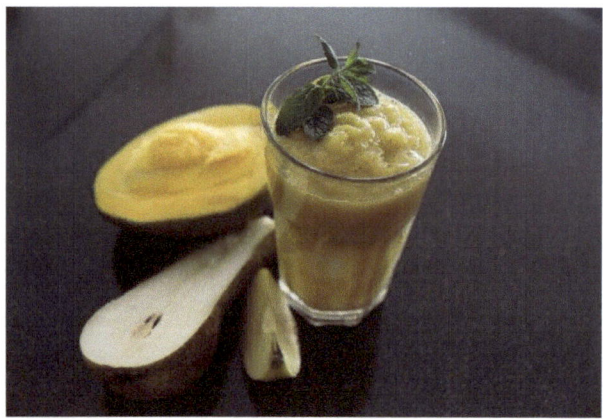

Kiwi Watercress Smoothie

- 2 sliced and chopped kiwis
- a handful of torn mint leaves
- 1 fresh lime juice
- 1 fresh orange juice, freshly squeezed or packed
- 50g watercress chopped

Whizz all fruit and vegetable ingredients together in a blender followed by the lime and orange juice.

Very Berry Smoothie

- 1 tablespoon honey
- 1 ½ cups of mixed berries (blueberries, mulberries, blackberries, strawberries)
- ¼ cup almond milk
- ½ cup ice cube
- 1 cup greek yogurt

Mix all ingredients in the blender until smooth.

Grape Dates Green Smoothie

- 1 cup sliced grapes
- 1 medium sized date
- 1/2 cup fresh spinach
- 1 cup coconut water

Mix all ingredients into the blender and blend until smooth and creamy.

Power Jumble Smoothie

- 1 cup cabbage greens, chopped thinly
- 1 cup pineapple juice
- 1 cup sliced carrots
- ½ cup mint leaves
- 1 freshly squeezed lemon juice
- 1 cup cherry tomatoes

Mix all ingredients into the blender and blend until smooth and creamy.

Banana Berry Smoothie

- 1 cup spinach
- 1 cup pure water
- 1cup sliced bananas
- 1 cup fresh blueberries

Mix all ingredients into the blender and blend until smooth and creamy.

Green Pumpkin Smoothie

- 1/3 cup pumpkin puree
- ½ cup coconut milk
- 1/3 cup plain yogurt
- ½ teaspoon cinnamon
- 2 ripe bananas, sliced
- 1 cup fresh spinach leaves

First, puree separately the pumpkin. When done, blend together with other fruits and vegetable ingredients.

Green Avocado Smoothie

- 1 cup spinach
- 1 ¼ cup soy milk
- ½ medium avocado, peeled and chopped
- ½ cup fresh mango
- 1 ripe banana
- ½ teaspoon honey

Mix all ingredients into the blender and blend until smooth and creamy.

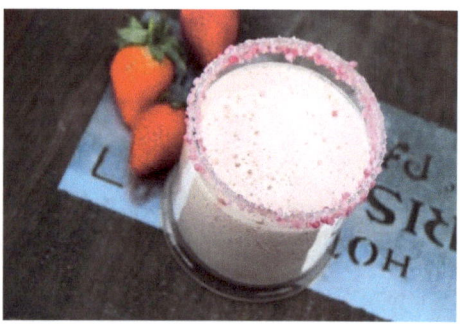

Berry Cauliflower Smoothie

- 1 tablespoon chia seeds
- 5 ripe bananas, sliced
- 1 ½ cups cauliflower
- 1 cup pure water
- 12 ounce fresh strawberries

Mix all ingredients into the blender and blend until smooth and creamy.

Pineapple Wheatgrass Smoothie

- 1 cup fresh pineapple, peeled and chopped
- ½ cold water
- 2 cups wheatgrass or wheatgrass juice
- 1 carrot, peeled and sliced
- 1 scoop wheatgrass powder
- 1 tablespoon lemon juice
- 1 tablespoon agave

Mix all ingredients into the blender and blend until smooth and creamy.

Avocado Sprout Smoothie

- 1 tablespoon fresh mint leaves
- dash of salt
- dash of cayenne pepper
- 1 cup of soy milk
- 1 tablespoon lime juice
- 1 medium-sized avocado, peeled and sliced
- 1 tablespoon honey
- ½ cup sprouts

Mix all ingredients into the blender and blend until smooth and creamy.

Amazing Sunflower Greens Smoothie

- 1 cup alfalfa
- 1 carrot, peeled and sliced
- 1 red apple, unpeeled and sliced
- 1 tablespoon agave
- 1 cup sunflower greens
- 1 cup kale

Mix all ingredients into the blender and blend until smooth and creamy.

Pineapple, Banana, and Kale Smoothie

- 1 ½ cup of sliced pineapple of medium size
- ½ cup coconut milk
- 2 cups hashed kale
- 1 full grown banana sliced into medium size

Add together 1 ½ cup of sliced pineapple, ½ cup coconut milk, 2 cups hashed kale and 1 sliced banana.

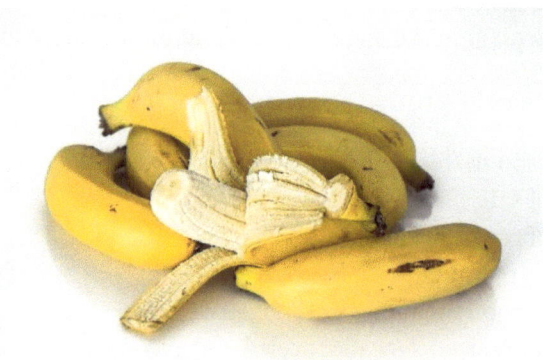

Ginger Power Smoothie

- 1 lemon, unpeeled and sliced
- 1 tablespoon ginger, unpeeled and sliced thinly
- 8 leaves of romaine lettuce, chopped
- 6 cups baby spinach, chopped
- 2 red apples, unpeeled and sliced
- 1/3 cup cucumber, unpeeled and sliced
- 2-3 garlic cloves, chopped thinly

Jumble all ingredients together leaving the garlic last to blend. Start with mixing 1 garlic clove first and adjust quantity as you feel appropriate to your taste.

CONCLUSION

This book provides you very useful information about Green Smoothies. You get to know about some best recipes of Smoothies and their benefits. Views and testimonials of different people are also mentioned in this book. You can read their personal experiences that would help you to develop your outlook on green smoothies. Green Smoothies are best for detoxification and weight loss purposes. You can try and enjoy the recipes mentioned above.

Thanks again for trusting the book!

About the Author

M. William

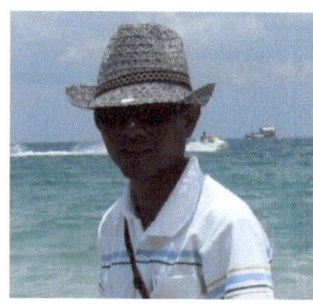

I have been writing articles dealing with the beauty, diet, weight loss and personal health for over 5 years more effectively through high quality web editorial and eBooks.

Thank you.

You contact M. William

Email: writingthai@gmail.com
Website: http://www.healthmay.com
Facebook: https://www.facebook.com/The10daygreensmoothiecleanse-699810736785103/
Google+ : https://plus.google.com/u/0/106858683551234517986/posts

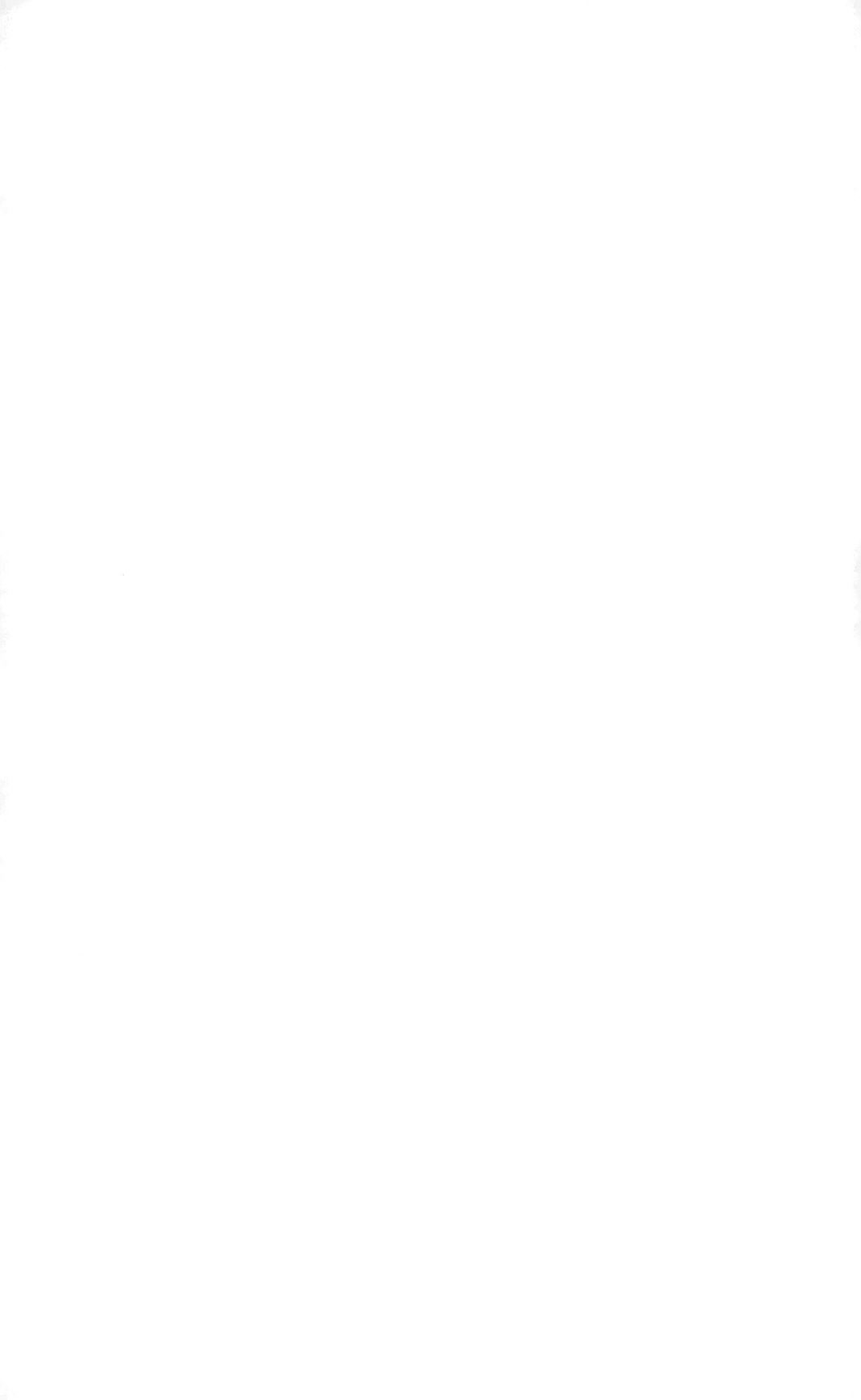

www.ingramcontent.com/pod-product-compliance
Lightning Source LLC
Chambersburg PA
CBHW050819290526
45792CB00001B/182